Penguin Health
Anorexia Nervosa

Robert Palmer was born in 1944 and educated at Warwick School, University College, and St George's Hospital Medical School, London. After doing postgraduate training in psychiatry, he went on to do research into anorexia nervosa and other psychosomatic disorders. He was lecturer at St Mary's Hospital Medical School, University of London, and in 1975 was appointed Senior Lecturer in Psychiatry at the new medical school of the University of Leicester.

Robert Palmer is married and has one daughter.

R. L. Palmer

ANOREXIA NERVOSA

A guide for sufferers and their families

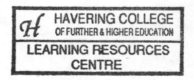

PENGUIN BOOKS

PENGUIN BOOKS

Published by the Penguin Group
27 Wrights Lane, London W8 5TZ, England
Viking Penguin Inc., 40 West 23rd Street, New York, New York 10010, USA
Penguin Books Australia Ltd, Ringwood, Victoria, Australia
Penguin Books Canada Ltd, 2801 John Street, Markham, Ontario, Canada L3R 1B4
Penguin Books (NZ) Ltd, 182–190 Wairau Road, Auckland 10, New Zealand

Penguin Books Ltd, Registered Offices: Harmondsworth, Middlesex, England

First published 1980
Second edition 1989
3 5 7 9 10 8 6 4 2

Made and printed in Great Britain by
Richard Clay Ltd, Bungay, Suffolk
Filmset in 10 on 12pt Sabon

Contents

Introduction and acknowledgements

I have written this book for two groups of people and for myself. Firstly, I wrote it for that mythical creature 'the interested general reader', although I am aware that the interest in this case may spring from painful personal experience of the illness in oneself or someone close. The book is not intended to be a handbook on what to do if you or your child has anorexia nervosa, but nevertheless I hope that it may help to make the disorder a little more comprehensible and perhaps a little less frightening than it might otherwise seem. Secondly, I wrote it for those who become professionally involved with anorexics without being specialists on the topic (for example, teachers, social workers and counsellors) as well as those working within the health services such as doctors, nurses, clinical psychologists and occupational therapists. Lastly, I wrote it for myself as a means of sorting out my own thinking about this puzzling disorder.

I have attempted to write in a way that is digestible, even by those whose intellectual diet is not usually medical or scientific. I have included a number of case histories or clinical sketches. In most of them I started to write with a particular person in mind but then changed some details so as to disguise the actual case. I do not wish to publish histories which could be identified in any way. If any of my patients read this book, they may recognize bits of themselves, but they will usually find that they are mixed with bits of other people! It follows that the case histories should be viewed as illustration, not as evidence. For convenience's sake, I have used a convention by which all anorexics are spoken of as female and all doctors as male.

No one should see this book as providing 'the truth' about anorexia nervosa. There is a danger that the specialist riding his hobby-horse will seem to know all the answers. His fellow experts realize how precarious his position is, but others may be fooled. The ideas put forward in this book are provisional. Many people reading the book may disagree greatly with my selection from the evidence and the interpretation which I describe. I sincerely hope that before long the model of anorexia nervosa which I favour will be improved or superseded by a better one. But this is the essence of scientific activity. The basis of clinical practice is to use creatively the current 'best buy' in understanding and thereby to help the patient. Furthermore, I would not wish to give the impression that the theory of anorexia nervosa put forward in this book is my own in the sense that it originated with me. It is, rather, my version of one of the current streams of thought on the disorder to which many workers have contributed, most notably Professor Arthur Crisp of St George's Hospital Medical School, London. Professor Crisp has done as much as anyone to explore and clarify the nature of anorexia nervosa. He was my mentor in these matters. I owe a great deal to him and the rest of the colleagues who worked at St George's in the early 1970s.

I also wish to thank those who contributed to the actual creation of the book, such as the friends and colleagues who read passages and made useful comments. Mrs June Shillitoe and Mrs Kim Brooks cheerfully bashed out page after page and their interpretation of my handwriting was almost always correct and when it was not, their version sometimes made better sense than my own. Penny Leach and Peter Wright of Penguin Books bullied me in the nicest possible way into changing some of my most cherished but most turgid passages into more acceptable prose. Somehow they combined precise criticism of parts with supportive enthusiasm for the whole. There are tricks in every trade. Lastly, it is almost customary to thank one's wife and say that without her the book would not have been written. Truly, Mary contributed a great deal, but I think that I could have written it without her; however, in the process life would have been infinitely more tedious.

R.L.P.
1980

In the introduction to the first edition of this book I emphasized the provisional nature of the ideas expressed in it and predicted, and even hoped for, change. It would be wrong to imply that the intervening seven or eight years have brought any dramatic breakthrough in the understanding or treatment of anorexia nervosa. However, enough change has occurred to make a substantially revised edition desirable. The changes of ideas and presentation are mainly shifts of emphasis rather than radical new insights, but have brought some parts of the puzzle together to make, perhaps, a little more sense. My own understanding of the disorder has been greatly enhanced by working with my colleagues at Leicester. Many have come and gone and have assisted substantially along the way but Pamela Marshall and Rhoda Oppenheimer have continued to make an enormous contribution for which I am truly grateful. The management of anorexia nervosa is usually a matter of teamwork, as is research. However, through necessity writing is a solo occupation; I hope that I have represented adequately the views of the team in which I work.

R.L.P.
Leicester 1987

1 · *The puzzle of anorexia nervosa*

A teenage girl gets on to a crowded bus. She sits down and starts to read a book. Next she opens a pack of gum and begins to chew. It is a hot summer day but she is well covered by a huge shirt and baggy jeans. However, her clothes fail to disguise her extreme thinness. Her cheeks are hollow, her complexion is pale and her eyes seem like islands of life in her tired and unhealthy face. She does not look at the other passengers, but they are looking at her. When she stands up and leaves the bus, they watch her go and then some begin to talk about her. More than one identifies her correctly as suffering from anorexia nervosa.

The words 'anorexia nervosa' are now quite widely known. Two or three decades ago this was not so. Then the disorder was often thought of as an esoteric rarity and mentioned only in the small print of medical textbooks. Today anorexia is discussed in popular programmes on the television and not uncommonly crops up in newspapers and in magazines. Most people have heard of the condition, although different people will think of it in widely differing ways. One person may have known a teenage girl who seemed to be deliberately attempting to mould herself into the shape of a 'slender' fashion model. Another may have been upset and worried by a neighbour who was clearly seriously ill. Likewise, the media may portray anorexia sometimes as an adolescent fad and sometimes as a mysterious killer disease, for which the boffins have yet to 'break through' to a cure. Few people know much about the nature of the disorder and many young people who are anorexic go unrecognized as such by their family and friends because their symptoms are not part of these popular pictures of the disorder. Furthermore, doctors receive little tuition in the condition and may not consider it except in obvious cases.

What is anorexia nervosa? How can the behaviour of the anorexic be understood? This book will describe the disorder and present some of the puzzles and problems which are encountered when trying to understand it.

The central features of anorexia nervosa

The word anorexia means loss of appetite. However, loss of appetite in the sense of never being hungry is not a central or necessary feature of anorexia nervosa. In fact, an anorexic may at times be very hungry. Nevertheless, she will characteristically behave as if she had lost her appetite since to eat normally would lead her to gain weight. Anorexia nervosa is essentially about weight rather than eating. A central feature of the disorder is *a body weight which is abnormally low* for the age, height and sex of the person. However, there are many other reasons why someone may be abnormally thin. What is more specific is the subject's *attitude to her weight*. Someone in a state of anorexia nervosa will not always be frank about her feelings, but when she is she will say that she is frightened of the thought of being heavier. She may suffer through being thin, but compared with putting on weight it is seen as the lesser evil. Professor Crisp of St George's Hospital Medical School, London, has coined the term 'weight phobia' to describe this attitude. A phobia is a morbid fear leading to the avoidance of that which is feared. The anorexic has a phobia of her normal body weight. Whether or not she is ready to admit this fear, the anorexic will behave in a way which leads her to become and then remain markedly thin and hence to avoid being at a normal weight. This determined and purposeful maintenance of thinness sets the anorexic apart. Other changes of behaviour and bodily function typically accompany the low body weight, notably cessation of menstruation, so called *secondary amenorrhoea*. Thus, the three central features of anorexia nervosa are an abnormally low body weight, an attitude and behaviour which tends to maintain this low weight (weight phobia) and other occurrences such as loss of periods which suggest a disordered physiology.

Of course, anorexia nervosa with weight phobia is not the only psychiatric state which may lead people to lose weight and eat oddly. Psychotic disorder with delusions about contamination of food, depression of mood with true loss of appetite, obsessional states and interpersonal difficulties with those who are involved in providing food, may all lead to states which closely resemble true anorexia nervosa, but the weight phobia will be absent. The term secondary anorexia nervosa is sometimes used to denote these states in contrast to the term primary anorexia nervosa which is reserved for the disorder with weight phobia. In this book, unless otherwise stated, the words anorexia nervosa will refer to primary anorexia nervosa rather than the range of secondary states.

The size of the problem

Anorexia nervosa can no longer be considered a rare disorder. It is increasingly recognized, talked about and studied. As an illustration, in 1945 three new articles on the subject appeared in world medical literature, in 1955 the number was seventeen and in 1965, it was twenty-five. By 1975 the annual rate of new publications had risen to sixty-eight, and by 1985 that total had more than doubled to 184 articles. Papers about the condition pour out from the United Kingdom and the rest of the developed world. While the general bulk of medical writing has also grown substantially in this forty-year period, this more than sixty-fold increase in articles is exceptional for a disease which has been recognized by the medical profession for many decades.

It is difficult to be certain whether all this attention has led to an increased rate of recognition, thus explaining the growing number of cases, or whether in fact the condition has become more common in recent years. Both have probably occurred. There have been a number of recent studies which have suggested that the disorder has become more prevalent. A report published in 1973 described three areas where careful registers had been kept over a number of years of cases from defined populations which presented to psychiatrists. One area was in London, one was in Scotland and one was in New York State; in each of these there was an increase in the number of cases over the period of study (Kendell *et al.*, 1973). Similarly, Dr May Duddle working in the Manchester University Student Health Service observed a marked rise in students presenting with the condition over the years from 1968 to 1971 when they constituted 11 per cent of referrals (Duddle, 1973). However, studies involving the counting of people presenting to medical services cannot distinguish a true increase in the disorder from an increase in the proportion of those with the condition who come to the attention of doctors. It is certain that not every sufferer seeks help, while some who do so may be wrongly diagnosed and thus remain undetected. Perhaps only a minority reaches specialist help. Nevertheless, these studies do indicate that the disorder may have truly increased in incidence over the last few years.

There can be no doubt that among some groups of young women and girls the disorder is at present quite common. A study of schoolgirls in seven private schools and two comprehensive schools in England showed that in the former, one girl in every hundred in the sixteen-and-over age group was suffering from the disorder. Interestingly, there seemed to be fewer cases in the comprehensive schools (Crisp, Palmer and Kalucy, 1976). Bearing in mind that perhaps a majority of sufferers are above school age, it would seem that in terms of numbers alone anorexia nervosa is a major health problem among adolescent girls and young women. While it would be over dramatic to talk in terms of a world-wide 'epidemic', anorexia nervosa is by no means a trivial condition and the number of cases now being reported throughout the developed world represents a considerable challenge.

There is something paradoxical in the fact that the problem of wilful starvation seems to occur most commonly in the richer countries of the world and perhaps among the better off within those countries. Caught at the other end of a world-wide system, many citizens of the Third World also starve. Their poverty may give them little choice of diet, and traditional proscriptions and preferences may narrow still further the range of foods which are eaten. In the developed world lack of choice is rarely the problem but, nevertheless, malnutrition, broadly defined, may not be uncommon. Many important diseases may be promoted by the food we eat. Thus arterial disease may be related to the over-consumption of certain animal fats, sugar certainly hastens the development of dental caries and various bowel disorders including cancer could be made more prevalent by diets low in fibre. Furthermore, obesity leads to both poor health and premature death. About a third of those men who are 20 per cent or more overweight are likely to die prematurely. Those who live at the wealthy end of the world's economy may succumb to the dangers of the 'rich' diets that are available to them or pushed upon them. Faced with a choice of diet we do not always choose wisely. However, the individual with anorexia nervosa seems to be making a more radical rejection of healthy eating. That she seems to choose to starve amid plenty makes her state more distressing and more puzzling. In the affluent part of the modern world anorexia nervosa stands out clearly from the background, and has recently received a great deal of attention; but it is not a 'new' condition.

Early medical descriptions

For over one hundred years, reports have appeared in the medical literature of people, mostly young women, who have lost a great deal of weight and become ill apparently because of a refusal to eat sufficient food. Indeed, fasting subjects have been a source of fascination and of study for many centuries (Morgan, 1977). However, the syndrome or clinical picture of anorexia nervosa was first described in the last century and although authors have emphasized different features, the central core has remained constant. Some of the earliest descriptions remain among the best.

The first detailed descriptions date from 1873. In that year two physicians, one English and one French, published independent accounts of the disorder. The Englishman, Sir William Withey Gull, was an eminent practitioner who treated the Prince of Wales when he had typhoid and who subsequently became a physician to Queen Victoria. He worked and indeed lived for many years at Guy's Hospital, London. Sir William was also an enthusiast for 'rescuing' prostitutes and his activities have recently led to speculation that he may have been Jack the Ripper (Knight, 1976).

Gull had mentioned the disorder in an address at Oxford in 1868, but his 1873 paper was devoted to it. The following is the first of two case histories included in Gull's paper 'as fair examples of the whole'. The account still serves as such.

Miss A., *aet.* 17, under the care of Mr Kelson Wright, of the Clapham Road, was brought to me on Jan. 17, 1866. Her emaciation was very great. It was stated that she had lost 33 lbs in weight. She was then 5 st. 12 lbs. Height, 5 ft 5 in.

Amenorrhoea for nearly a year. No cough. Respirations throughout chest everywhere normal. Heart sounds normal. Resp. 12; pulse, 56. No vomiting nor diarrhoea. Slight constipation. Complete anorexia for animal food, and almost complete anorexia for everything else. Abdomen shrunk and flat, collapsed. No abnormal pulsations of aorta. Tongue clean. Urine normal. Slight deposit of phosphates on boiling. The condition was one of simple starvation. There was but slight variation in her condition, though observed at intervals of three or four months ... The case was regarded as one of simple anorexia.

Various remedies were prescribed – the preparations of cinchona, the bichloride of mercury, syrup of the iodide of iron, syrup of the phosphate of iron, citrate of quinine and iron, etc, but no perceptible effect followed their administration. The diet also was varied, but without any effect upon the appetite. Occasionally for a day or two the appetite was voracious, but this was very rare and exceptional. The patient complained of no pain, but was restless and active. This was in fact a striking expression of the nervous state, for it seemed hardly possible that a body so wasted could undergo the exercise which seemed agreeable. There was some peevishness of temper, and a feeling of jealousy. No account could be given of the exciting cause.

Miss A. remained under my observation from Jan. 1866 to March 1868, when she had much improved, and gained weight from 82 to 128 lbs. The improvement from this time continued, and I saw no more of her medically.

The picture given by Sir William Gull is clear and recognizable as that of anorexia nervosa, a name he coined. He goes on to give his views on the nature of the disorder.

The want of appetite is, I believe, due to a morbid mental state. I have not observed in these cases any gastric disorder to which the want of appetite could be referred. I believe, therefore, that its origin is central and not peripheral. That mental states may destroy appetite is notorious, and it will be admitted that young women at the ages named are specially obnoxious to mental perversity. We might call the state hysterical without committing ourselves to the etymological value of the word, or maintaining that the subjects of it have the common symptoms of hysteria. I prefer, however, the more general term, 'nervosa', since the disease occurs in males as well as females, and is probably rather central than peripheral. The importance of discriminating such cases in practice is obvious; otherwise prognosis will be erroneous, and treatment misdirected.

The account published by Gull's French contemporary, Dr E. C. Lasegue, is perhaps richer but less clear cut and contains more speculation. In particular Lasegue is concerned to place the disorder as a variant of hysteria. This protean concept was often evoked as an explanation of illness at the time. However, some of his comments are worth quoting. Thus he writes about the subject's attitude to her condition:

> What dominates in the mental condition of the hysterical patient is, above all, the state of quietude – I might almost say a condition of contentment truly pathological. Not only does she not sigh for recovery, but she is not ill-pleased with her condition, notwithstanding all the unpleasantness it is attended with. In comparing this satisfied assurance to the obstinacy of the insane I do not think I am going too far. Compare this with all the other forms of anorexia, and observe how different they are.

He observes the relationship between the patient and those around her.

> The anorexia gradually becomes the sole object of preoccupation and conversation. The patient thus gets surrounded by a kind of atmosphere, from which there is no escape during the entire day. Friends join counsels with relatives, each contributing to the common stock, according to the nature of his disposition or the degree of his affection. Now, there is another most positive law that hysteria is subject to the influence of the surrounding medium, and that the disease becomes developed and condensed so much the more as the circle within which revolve the ideas and sentiments of the patient becomes more narrowed.

Anyone who has lived with anorexia or an anorexic person will know what Dr Lasegue meant!

The puzzle of anorexia nervosa

Anorexia nervosa is difficult to understand, since for most people regular feeding is routine. If it is disrupted, hunger quickly drives them to eat. The difficulty of even minor slimming for many people is evidence enough of this. How then can the extreme behaviour of the anorexic be understood? An anorexic is clearly not well physically, but her attitude and frame of mind are also unusual, and could be construed as morbid. Is it best to think of the root of the problem in psychological or physical terms? There is no certain answer, and over the years since the time of Gull and Lasegue, various explanations have been put forward. Both of these earliest authorities favoured the view that the state was to be understood as arising in the mind: a mental disorder which leads to extreme physical consequences simply because the sufferer behaves as she does and deprives her body of adequate nourishment. However, a largely physical interpretation is also possible. Appetite, eating, mood, sexual feeling and menstruation may all be influenced by a part of the brain known as the hypothalamus and it is plausible that malfunction of the hypothalamus could be the primary disorder, and that the complicated emotional tangles which are often so evident within and around the anorexic subject could be secondary. As will be discussed in Chapter 4, the hypothalamus controls the pituitary gland, which is involved with other endocrine (hormone-producing) glands. In 1914, M. Simmonds described a state of emaciation and amenorrhoea which was a result of physical disease of the pituitary gland. For a time, therefore, there was some confusion between Simmonds' disease and anorexia nervosa. It has been suggested that many anorexics were misdiagnosed until clear criteria for differentiating the two disorders became available (Dally, 1969). Even when this particular problem was clarified there was still no clear consensus as to the nature of primary anorexia nervosa. Many confusing views remain; some more clearly based on evidence and others apparently the result of speculation alone. Anorexia nervosa is still a puzzle. However, parts of the puzzle seem to have fallen into place recently and most investigators would now acknowledge that both psychological and somatic 'pieces' are required to make up the more satisfactory explanations.

If problems understanding the disorder persist, there are also difficulties in knowing how to approach its treatment. Here again both purely psychological and purely physical interventions have been advocated in the past and are still practised. Today most authorities favour treatment programmes which include elements of both, although it would be quite wrong to suggest that there is agreement about what technique or combination of techniques is best. Chapter 6 reviews the range of treatment which may be offered.

For the parents and others who are close to a person who is trapped within the condition, the puzzle of anorexia nervosa may resemble a maze from which there seems to be no escape. For them the difficulty in understanding the disorder is experienced as a distressing failure to empathize with a young person who seems to have abandoned her previous course through life in favour of a 'one-track' preoccupation with weight and eating, which at best may seem eccentric and at worst is clearly self-destructive. There can be few more difficult experiences for parents than to see their child wasting away while refusing the offers of food which seem such a tantalizingly simple solution to the problem. It is often suggested that the young people who fall ill with anorexia nervosa come from families with more than their fair share of interpersonal and other problems. If this is true then the anguish of the parents may well be the greater for it.

At the centre of this web of uncertainty and doubt, the anorexic subject exists in a state of painful puzzlement. For her, it is her own body and behaviour which have changed for reasons which even she does not fully understand. She feels that she has no room to move. She is squashed into a narrow range of feelings and behaviour by strong forces which she does not understand but which are none the less frightening as they arise unequivocally from within herself. She may or may not acknowledge the tragic absurdity of her position when seen through the eyes of others, but it will be the dictates of her fears and feelings that will almost always prevail when she is confronted with the possibility of weight gain. The term 'gut reaction' seems to be particularly appropriate here and the 'gut reactions' of the anorexic are stronger than the appeals of even her own common sense. A person may be able to walk with confidence and ease along a narrow plank placed on the ground; the same walk would seem terrifying or even impossible if the plank were to be suspended in the air, even if it represented the escape route from a fire or other calamity. The simple act of eating must often have something of the same frightening quality for the anorexic.

2 · What is anorexia nervosa?

This chapter attempts to describe the symptoms, signs, behavioural patterns and features which occur in people with anorexia nervosa. It is concerned with description rather than explanation, inasmuch as these can be separated.

Defining characteristics

Doctors diagnose anorexia nervosa on the basis of the patient's history and clinical features rather than by relying upon tests or investigations. The presence of the disorder cannot be precisely confirmed in the way that an infectious disease or a cancer might be demonstrated by finding characteristic organisms or abnormal cells. What then are the defining characteristics of the disorder? There have been a number of attempts to define diagnostic criteria clearly. Professor Russell of the Institute of Psychiatry, University of London, outlined in 1970 three essential features which may be summarized as follows:

1. Behaviour leading to a marked loss of body weight. A studied avoidance of foods considered to be of a fattening nature. Often but not invariably the subject resorts to additional devices which ensure a loss of weight: self-induced vomiting or purgation, or excessive exercise. Occasional bouts of overeating may occur.

2. An endocrine disorder (disorder of hormones) which manifests itself clinically by cessation of menstruation in females.

3. A morbid fear of becoming fat which may be fully expressed by the subject or may be more explicit in her behaviour. To safeguard herself against what she calls 'losing control' – meaning not being able to stop eating – she strives to remain abnormally thin.

These criteria are straightforward, clear and useful. For particular purposes, however, it may be necessary to have more sharply defined rules which produce a clear, if arbitrary distinction between 'cases' and 'non-cases'. Some kinds of research demand this approach. Such a definition of anorexia nervosa has been produced by a team of psychiatrists in St Louis in the United States (Feighner, Robins and Guze, 1972). It will serve both as a contrast with the criteria quoted above and as a useful summary of many of the important features of the disorder.

1. Age of onset prior to twenty-five.

2. Anorexia with accompanying weight loss of at least 25 per cent of original body weight.

3. A distorted, implacable attitude towards eating, food, or weight that overrides hunger, admonitions, reassurance, and threats.

4. No known medical illness that could account for the anorexia and weight loss.

5. No other known psychiatric disorder with particular reference to primary affective disorders, schizophrenia, obsessive-compulsive and phobic neuroses.

6. At least two of the following: amenorrhoea, lanugo (excessive, fine body hair), bradycardia (slow pulse-rate), periods of over-activity, episodes of bulimia (uncontrolled gorging of food), vomiting.

It is important to note that the majority of cases diagnosed on one of these sets of criteria would undoubtedly be diagnosed in the same way by the other set. Many people hover on the borderland of anorexia nervosa and, therefore, present difficulties of diagnosis or definition. Both sets, however, offer minimal outlines of anorexia nervosa. The rest of this chapter will attempt to expand upon these outlines and will emphasize the way in which people who are properly described as suffering from primary anorexia nervosa may differ from each other as well as the ways in which they may appear the same.

Who develops anorexia nervosa?

It is usually uncertain why any particular individual develops primary anorexia nervosa. Nevertheless, it is clear that the risk of
doing so varies between different sections of the population. It is
possible in broad terms to predict what sort of people are most
likely to fall ill in this way. This is, of course, useful knowledge in
its own right; furthermore, clues obtained from studying the dis-
tribution of a disorder in a population can often help in developing
ideas about its nature and causes. This kind of study is part of the
medical science of epidemiology. The detection of the important
link between smoking and lung cancer is an example of epidem-
iological research.

Age and sex are two factors which seem to have a major influence
on the risk of developing anorexia nervosa. The vast majority of
cases are female; indeed, in most series which have been described,
males account for less than one in ten. This skew is interesting
because while many conditions are commoner in one sex than the
other, in few is the inequality of risk so great. What makes females
so relatively vulnerable and males so relatively resistant to the
disorder? However, while this seems to be the norm, primary anorexia nervosa with phobia *does* occur quite unequivocally in
males. The hormonal disorder in these young men would seem to
resemble that which occurs in female anorexics although, of
course, the gross evidence of it by the cessation of menstruation
is not available. It may be that anorexia nervosa is sometimes
misdiagnosed in males because doctors do not consider the possibility when confronted by a man, but it is unlikely that this is
the main reason for the scarcity of reports of the disorder in
men.

Most anorexics are, therefore, female and most of these are girls
and young women in their teens and twenties. In two large British
series (Dally, 1969; Crisp and Stonehill, 1971) the commonest age
at which weight loss began was fifteen, although the age of onset
ranged from ten or eleven to the third decade or beyond. There is
usually some delay between the onset of the disorder and the time
when the anorexic seeks help. She will often be a most reluctant
patient.

Almost all cases of primary anorexia nervosa occur after puberty and before the menopause. A few children seem to develop the condition before any clear evidence of the onset of puberty and more than a few at just about the time of their first period. However, some reported cases in younger children may be more akin to neurotic problems with food refusal than true anorexia nervosa with weight phobia. Likewise, psychiatric states with predominant weight loss after the fourth decade are more commonly not true primary anorexia nervosa, although it would be rash to say that the disorder cannot occur at the menopause or even beyond. At least one convincing case has been reported in a woman of fifty-one years of age at onset (Kellett, Trimble and Thorley, 1976).

The most typical anorexic is, then, a girl in her late teenage years. While other factors are probably of importance, it is likely that both the age and sex distributions of the condition are related to the frequency of slimming. Teenage girls very frequently diet to lose weight with the idea of improving their figures, and indeed to be unconcerned about such matters is the exception (Nylander, 1971). Slimming at this age is commonly not the lone struggle which it may often be in older people but is rather a concern which is shared by a girl with her peers. Teachers relay anecdotes of whole classes becoming weight conscious and participating in slimming crazes. Adolescence is commonly a time of personal uncertainty and self-consciousness. It is perhaps understandable that the teenage girl growing up in our society should feel that moulding her body is a way to self-improvement. Most girls would like to look like the models on the hoardings, but most girls do not. The teenage magazines cater to this concern. On the other hand, it is much less common for boys of the same age to seek to lose weight and indeed many are concerned with increasing their bulk and improving their physique. Of the many girls and young women who go on slimming diets, only a few will develop anorexia nervosa. Nevertheless, the prevalence of slimming behaviour may crucially affect the number of people who develop the disorder, just as the extent of alcohol consumption in a population as a whole may influence the number of people who develop drinking problems.

A third factor which may influence risk is social class. The risk seems to be greater in the 'higher' classes. However, whenever such a pattern of disease is observed, it is necessary to consider that it may reflect a bias of observation or presentation to doctors. Perhaps anorexic subjects from poorer backgrounds are relatively neglected and are, therefore, under-represented in published accounts of the disorder. This possibility cannot be entirely dismissed, but on the whole it does seem probable that anorexia nervosa is more common in the middle and upper classes. Again a higher rate of slimming and concern about weight may in part explain this tendency, for although obesity is more common among working-class women, it has been, at least until recently, much less worried about. Just a few decades ago to be plump was evidence of a degree of financial security which was beyond the reach of everyone. Perhaps the shadow of hunger is only just passing from the attitudes of the present generation. Nevertheless, obesity is undoubtedly an important antecedent of anorexia nervosa, and a significant proportion of anorexics are found to have been overweight.

While age, sex, social class and weight are all related to the risk of developing anorexia nervosa, they are rather crude predictors and would be of little value if used alone to identify potential anorexics. Have any additional risk factors been identified? Clinical experience suggests further items, but their nature and the evidence upon which they are based are less clear cut and reliable. It seems likely that the young person who develops anorexia nervosa may well have been experiencing more than the usual difficulty in negotiating the tricky transition from child to adult even before she fell ill. However, such difficulties are not specific and may reflect either vulnerability of personality or problems in circumstances or both. Likewise, there is good anecdotal evidence that, in the experience of anorexic subjects, food and eating, and weight and activity are frequently highly emotional topics before the disorder itself becomes established. For instance, the parents may work in the food industry or may themselves have unusually strong views about diet or weight. Sometimes these strong views arise because of the presence or a past history of other definite weight disorders in the family. Such family traditions may be both powerful and unusual. A child growing up in such a family may develop views on the meaning of appetite, weight, indulgence and so on which are markedly odd. It is not difficult to see how such views might increase the risk of falling ill. In addition, there is clear evidence that anorexia nervosa runs in families. It is uncertain whether this reflects the working of family tradition and atmosphere or the manifestation of a genetically transmitted vulnerability, though on balance the former seems more likely. However, there is some recent evidence that supports the idea of a genetic factor. Identical (monozygotic) twins have been shown to have a higher degree of concordance for eating disorder than non-identical (dyzygotic) twins (Crisp, Hall and Holland, 1985). Nevertheless, even if such a genetic factor does play a part, the nature of the vulnerability which is thus transmitted is unclear.

In what way do people enter the condition?

In order to enter the state of anorexia nervosa, a person must lose weight. The majority set out to do so deliberately because rightly or wrongly they feel that they are too fat. Some are indeed overweight. The prevalence of the condition seems to vary with that of slimming behaviour.

A person who sets out to lose weight may do so by cutting down the amount of all foods eaten or more commonly may selectively avoid foods which are thought to be especially 'fattening'. This usually means carbohydrate-rich foods and fatty foods. Thus starchy items like bread, potatoes, cakes and so on are dropped from the diet, as are fried foods and fatty meats. For most people dieting to lose weight is a struggle. Most dieters 'cheat' or give up before they lose all the weight which they had intended to shed. For those who do reach their intended weight there is a measure of satisfaction, although for some the price of continuing trimness is continuing vigilance and a process of re-education of eating habits. By contrast the anorexic-to-be may find slimming easy and rewarding from the start or at least discover that in a sense she is good at it. Characteristically she ends up by overshooting her intended weight and continuing to 'slim' despite the fact that she has already done so. In many cases, however, it seems that she has started out behaving like and with the same intentions of the ordinary slimmer. Something goes wrong and the slimming behaviour is inappropriately prolonged.

Sarah was the only child of rather elderly parents who were both somewhat obese. She had been plump from infancy and by the time she was sixteen she weighed 11 stones (70 kg). She was used to being called 'fatty' or 'the lump' at school and was always embarrassed when she had to change for games. She was a keen horsewoman and had had some success in competition. Her occasional attempts at dieting became more determined after she came to the conclusion that her increasing weight was becoming a handicap for her riding. She dieted with the encouragement of her parents and set out to lose 2 stones (12·7 kg). She passed this weight after less than three months, but continued to avoid fattening foods. After a further three months she weighed less than 7 stones (44·5 kg) and was unequivocally in a state of anorexia nervosa.

Anorexic girls often report some particular event or comment about weight which seems to have set them on the path that leads to the disorder. Often a parent or friend has teased them about being fat or perhaps about their appetite. It is difficult to be sure how truly significant these events are. Doubtless many plump young people have similar experiences, set out to lose weight with a similar resolve but either do not succeed in slimming or lose an appropriate amount of weight and then stop.

Christine was a 20-year-old student at university who, in common with many of her friends, decided to diet for cosmetic reasons even though she was only marginally over-weight. She was especially concerned about the shape of her hips and thighs. She had been rather unhappy for a number of reasons, and, in particular, a relationship with a boyfriend was going badly. Almost to her surprise she found that she was able to control her eating without much difficulty and before long eating any substantial amount gave her a feeling of being 'bloated'. On the other hand the sensation of 'emptiness' and of suppressed hunger gave her a 'good, clean feeling'. Her flatmates confronted her after they had seen her undressed when her weight had fallen to 6½ stones (41 kg).

This sense of satisfaction arising from the suppression of hunger is frequently reported by anorexic subjects and it is often experienced from the beginning. Perhaps in some way self-denial is especially rewarding for them.

Anorexia nervosa is sometimes described as 'the slimmers' disease' and clearly this name is appropriate to a degree. However, a minority of subjects enter the condition following a loss of weight which has occurred for reasons other than deliberate slimming. Thus a young person may lose weight because of physical illness and then fail to resume eating. Again the sensations associated with emptiness and low weight may come to be viewed positively and the feeling of a full stomach and possible weight gain come to seem undesirable or frightening. The result is still an avoidance of weight gain and of patterns of eating which might lead to it. It is possible that psychiatric disorder with diminished appetite or food refusal leading to weight loss may also sometimes evolve into true anorexia nervosa with weight phobia. Thus a depressed adolescent girl who loses her appetite may lose weight and then somehow become 'caught' by the weight loss and its consequences. Again the outcome may be a state of weight phobia which outlasts or even helps to resolve the depressed mood.

Once a young person has reached a markedly low weight, she will find herself in a clearly changed position and one that has disadvantages. However, her awareness of the changes and of their disadvantages may be concealed from those around her or even in some ways from herself. It would seem that her experience is dominated rather by a sense of relative control, safety or even triumph, although this is felt to be precarious and is threatened by any act which might lead to weight gain. The preservation of her new position against change or the threat of change becomes a central preoccupation which tends to distort other interests, concerns and relationships. The extent to which this becomes an absolute preoccupation varies, but in the extreme case the current position is never enough and weight loss progresses until it becomes life-threatening. More usually a kind of equilibrium is reached with a body weight which is 20 to 30 per cent below average.

Established anorexia nervosa

The anorexic established in this new position is changed both in body and behaviour, while her approach to personal relationships and her view of her world have also altered. However, to those around her the changes in her body weight and eating behaviour will be most evident. As was suggested above, the low body weight can be extreme but it may be less noticeable if the anorexic seeks to conceal it by wearing loose-fitting clothes, many layers of jumpers or other garments which hide her body contours. Parents and others often report the shock and surprise which they feel when they first see the person undressed and her emaciation is revealed. Such an event may often lead to the 'emergency' presentation to medical care of a subject who has, in fact, been in a state of anorexia nervosa for months or even years.

Patterns of eating in established anorexia nervosa may take two broad forms. The more common pattern is usually known as *abstinent anorexia nervosa*. Almost every anorexic begins with this pattern and many continue to behave in this way throughout their illness. Some, however, may develop other behaviour patterns as time passes.

The eating behaviour of the abstinent anorexic resembles ordinary slimming occurring in the inappropriate context of someone whose body weight is abnormally low. She works hard at limiting her diet and weight even though she is already very thin. Typically she will avoid all foods which she considers to be fattening, particularly foods which are high in carbohydrate. However, she may allow herself to eat substantial amounts of bulky but low calorie foods such as celery, crispbread or cottage cheese. Sometimes her diet will come to be not only very small in amount but also quite eccentric in its constituent foods. A few anorexics turn yellow through eating large numbers of carrots but little else. The whole gamut of slimming activity may be present although it often seems charged with a frantic force which is absent when slimming is a more understandable response to true obesity. What to the commonplace slimmer may be a struggle or a chore, to the anorexic may seem a source of morbid fascination. Calories are counted, single sausages are slowly grilled, lettuce leaves are selected with care, bran is eaten dry and slimming magazines are 'devoured'.

The anorexic will usually avoid eating with others at conventional mealtimes and her own meals, such as they are, may either be eaten in odd moments or in a ritualistic way at the same time and in the same circumstances each day. In terms of the total calorific value of food eaten, an abstinent anorexic will characteristically exist on an average daily intake of under 1,000 calories, compared with the norm of two or three times this amount.

The anorexic is struggling to keep up her position of abstinence in the face of not only her sensations of hunger but also the demands of a truly undernourished body. Although her behaviour resembles normal slimming, the context is quite different. Most anorexics will initially deny that they are hungry. Some probably do truly lose their appetite, but most will admit later that they experienced a strong desire to eat. Many sufferers become preoccupied with food. They are, for instance, eager to prepare meals for others which they will not eat themselves. Similarly, most anorexics have some lapses and eat more from time to time; when the iron self-control breaks, an eating binge may follow. At times, the amount of food eaten during one episode may be very large. It seems that for some individuals the struggle to control their weight by abstinence alone becomes too much and they find additional means. One may guess that these individuals are those in whom the hunger drive is greatest or the control of impulses is least developed. It is these subjects who go on to the *second broad pattern of eating behaviour* which is characterized by *overeating, self-induced vomiting* and often by the *abuse of laxatives and other drugs*. This pattern is known as *bulimic anorexia* or *bulimia nervosa* (Russell, 1979). In general, the establishment of this pattern is not a good sign (Casper *et al.*, 1980; Garfinkel, Moldofsky and Garner, 1980).

Vomiting will often start when an abstinent anorexic feels bloated and uncomfortable after she has, for once, 'let go' and eaten more than usual. She then vomits to relieve the discomfort and perhaps also the guilt which she feels about having indulged her appetite. Later, however, she may realize that vomiting is a kind of insurance policy against the effect of overeating because it interferes with the otherwise inevitable link between eating and weight. The fear of weight gain then no longer serves as a brake upon the impulse to eat and overeating may become both substantial and regular. The vomiting which started as a response to unwelcome inner feelings may become premeditated. Anorexic subjects often develop a considerable facility for vomiting. An individual may come to be able to vomit at will without, for instance, the need to stick her fingers down her throat.

Sometimes vomiting may allow the person to return to a more regular pattern of eating while avoiding weight gain. Thus some subjects may achieve a kind of stability combined with an apparently unremarkable diet. Two or three meals are eaten each day but each is vomited up again in secret shortly afterwards. It is possible for this pattern to continue for months or even years and yet for the anorexic to conceal her vomiting successfully from those near to her. Certainly some women with 'mysterious' thinness and 'mysterious' amenorrhoea accompanied by an apparently good appetite and diet are chronic covert vomiters. However, the stability of this pattern is more apparent than real since the subject is now involved in a balancing act. On the one hand, her eating behaviour may be linked to a routine of social expectations but is always more or less disrupted by impulses to overeat. On the other hand, she must vomit up sufficient of what she eats to keep her weight down but not so much as to render herself physically ill. Not surprisingly the seesaw usually begins to wobble and only in a few cases can a kind of fragile stability be maintained for long. Sometimes the balance swings in favour of weight gain which may provide the subject with the opportunity for recovery. Unfortunately it is more usual for her to panic as her weight increases and she will drastically cut back her food intake once more. Even chronic vomiters have times when they return to a predominantly abstinent pattern. However, the temptation to eat and then vomit is seldom resisted for long.

Although regular eating and regular vomiting may sometimes allow a kind of balance, the change from the abstinent mode to the overeating and vomiting mode more often leads to a marked loss of physical and emotional stability. The seesaw pitches more and more wildly and the anorexic finds herself in an increasingly frantic and chaotic state. The impulse to eat may become extreme and the preoccupation with food overwhelming. Extraordinary amounts of food of all kinds may be eaten in binges which go on until the stomach can take no more and copious vomiting follows. The food which is eaten during these binges usually includes all the fattening carbohydrate-rich foods which are avoided in periods of abstinence. Cream cakes by the plateful, whole loaves of bread, packets of sweets, biscuits and quantities of cheese are eaten rapidly and avidly but with little pleasure. Guilt and self-disgust mount as the abdomen swells and only vomiting brings relief and a brief respite.

Sometimes feeding behaviour becomes bizarre. A young woman from a financially secure background may search through dustbins for edible scraps. Another may steal food from shops. Such shoplifting is often understandable as a reflection of the dominating preoccupation with food, together with the impulsive nature of the appetite. The cost of supporting the habit of recurrent bulimia can resemble or even exceed the cost of the addiction of an alcoholic. Even where the chaos is contained within the home it can still be both surprising and disruptive.

Angela was the 22-year-old daughter of a retired naval officer. She had been anorexic for six years and had been overeating and vomiting regularly for five years. She weighed about 7 stones (44·5 kg) on average, but her weight ranged widely and erratically in response to her chaotic eating pattern. Two months before presentation to treatment she had been discovered stealing money from her grandmother's purse in order to buy food. A family crisis followed in which she told her parents for the first time about her vomiting. Subsequently her behaviour became increasingly uncontrolled. She would eat and then vomit any food which was available, cooked or uncooked, palatable or rotting. Her mother described how having placed a cake in the oven she returned after a few minutes to find her daughter on her knees scooping the cake mixture into her mouth with her bare hands.

Such extreme behaviour often makes the anorexic feel very anxious and out of control and she may actually plead for external control and, for instance, may ask for admission to hospital. Unfortunately her apparent motivation for radical change often disappears when she has recovered her aplomb and finds herself in a situation where she is expected to eat, has no opportunity for vomiting and is thus faced with the prospect of weight gain.

Vomiting is one method by which the link between diet and weight can be disrupted, but there are at least two others which anorexic subjects employ from time to time. Firstly, an anorexic may take increasing quantities of *laxatives*. Relative constipation is common in abstinent anorexia. This is hardly surprising because the intake of food is so low. An individual may get into the habit of laxative-taking through the self-treatment of such constipation. However, both the logic and the emotional tone of excessive purgation may prove tempting, especially where overeating has resulted in abdominal swelling and discomfort. To a young person who feels bloated and self-indulgent, a handful of laxative tablets may offer the prospect of both physical and mental catharsis. As with vomiting, regular laxative abuse can contribute to a vicious circle as it not only provides escape from the consequences of past indulgence but may make future bingeing more likely. If laxatives are to be employed the doses used are enough to induce diarrhoea; one or two extra tablets are simply not sufficient. Anorexic subjects for whom laxative abuse has become a central feature of their condition may take as many as fifty tablets per day. However, despite the belief held by some anorexic subjects that laxatives are an essential slimming aid, there is no evidence that this method is an effective means of weight control (Lacey and Gibson, 1985). The price of this drug abuse may be high in terms of discomfort, pain and ill health. Although a few subjects seem to experience relatively less discomfort than might be expected, many put up with colicky abdominal pain, anal soreness and even faecal incontinence. The desperation of such young people is evident in the extent to which they continue such gross over-purgation in spite of the suffering it brings. However, bodies must be less tolerant than minds as chronic laxative abuse usually leads to considerable metabolic disorder.

Diuretic drugs make up the second group which may be abused by anorexics in their struggle with their weight. Diuretics influence the fluid balance of the body by increasing the volume of urine which is passed. They are widely prescribed for heart failure and other conditions in which the body has a tendency to accumulate excessive fluid. Swelling of the legs due to fluid retention may occasionally occur after bulimia or when the body is low in protein and anorexics suffering from these complaints may be prescribed diuretics. A large dose of diuretics can cause a dramatic drop in weight which is most gratifying to the weight phobic. Such a loss is, of course, composed solely of fluid and is transient except where there had been abnormal fluid retention previously. If the weight loss is to be maintained, more diuretics are required and a state of chronic dehydration and biochemical imbalance follows. Once again the physical consequences can be serious.

It is difficult to be certain how frequently the different types of eating behaviour occur in individuals as there is considerable overlap between the groups. Initially, almost all subjects show an abstinent pattern usually as a prolongation of slimming behaviour. Moreover, many predominantly abstinent anorexics occasionally overeat while most overeaters have periods of self-starvation. Chronic overeating and vomiting or purgation tend to develop as complications of the abstinent mode. Both patterns may be associated with an overall disturbance of health and well-being ranging from the relatively less severe complications to the life-threatening. Nevertheless, in general the pattern which is characterized by overeating, together with some compensatory mechanism such as vomiting or excessive purgation, tends to be less stable, is associated with serious physical complications, is more difficult to treat and is more likely to become chronically prolonged. In most series of patients, persistent vomiters form at least one quarter of the total. Abusers of laxatives and diuretics are rather less common.

Whatever the predominant pattern of behaviour, the core of established primary anorexia nervosa remains the subject's fear of regaining a normal weight, and her efforts to avoid doing so. Many of the other characteristic changes in behaviour can be understood as the consequences of this core. Thus many anorexic subjects are surprisingly active. The anorexic's tendency to remain active and to exercise her body even when it is emaciated has been commented on since the time of the first descriptions of the disorder. Lasegue wrote in 1873:

> so far from muscular power being diminished, this abstinence tends to increase the aptitude for movement. The patient feels more light and active, rides on horseback, receives and pays visits and is able to pursue a fatiguing life in the world without perceiving the lassitude she would at other times have complained of.

Not all anorexic subjects are over-active, but some take activity to extremes by rarely sitting down, doing strenuous exercises, and going for runs even when their appearance would suggest they are on the point of collapse. When confined to bed some may continue to perform isometric muscle exercises under the blankets! Again, the early writers had observed the difficulty in imposing inactivity on anorexic subjects. Writing in 1929, Pierre Janet quotes a Dr Wallet as having written the following in a case description published in 1892.

The patient is exceedingly fond of long walks. As she is growing thinner with enormous rapidity, they are forbidden her. She then begins to walk, from morning to night, up and down the little garden of the house, which was likewise forbidden her. Then she plays all day at shuttlecock. It is prescribed that she stay in her room; there she gives herself up to violent gymnastic exercises. Even in bed she goes on with her gambols and somersaults.

Such subjects may be preoccupied with the concept of 'fitness', which, for them, is closely related to 'thinness', and as with 'thinness' it has come to be loaded with unusual importance and extra meaning. In spite of their apparently unusual capacity for physical exertion, it would probably be a mistake to view this as evidence of any special physical toughness; rather it is an indicator of their determination to be active in spite of the state of their physical health. Certainly, the anorexic may push herself to the point of collapse; such a crisis is another way in which a long-standing case may present to medical care as an emergency. The activity of the anorexic can be understood perhaps in two ways. Firstly, as a direct consequence of her weight phobia and the belief that exercise will help to 'burn off calories'. Secondly, it may be that she is experiencing the force of a basic biological urge often shown by half-starved animals which characteristically keep on the move. Presumably such behaviour carries an advantage when food is scarce and must be sought out. Likewise, there seems to be a biological link between sleep and nutrition which may have had survival value in the course of evolution. The sleep of the anorexic subject is usually disturbed and she will tend to wake early although she does not always find this a problem or complain about it (Crisp, Stonehill and Fenton, 1971).

Physical over-activity may also serve to distract the sufferer's attention from her hunger. Mental activity can also serve this purpose. When a girl moves into a state of anorexia nervosa she may change her pattern of interests markedly, but the change is usually a narrowing. If she is at school or a student her studies may come to be her only preoccupation; other, that is, than weight and eating.

Amanda was a 16-year-old border at a girls' public school well known for its high academic standards. She was intelligent and able, and tended to keep up with her class although her performance was usually no more than 'average' in this highly academic setting. She became anorexic early in her O-level year and subsequently began to spend more and more time studying. Half-way through the spring term she was sent home because of her physical state but continued to follow a self-imposed programme of study and revision involving over fourteen hours of work each day. She would allow herself one half-hour of television watching, one brief walk and some time to prepare for herself what little food she would eat. Any attempt by her parents and others to disrupt this pattern was met with anger and tears.

In such cases it is usual for academic success to be central to the family's sense of what it is to be a 'good' daughter, but the extremes to which the anorexic may take her studying can upset even the most demanding parents. Furthermore, although complex interpretations involving the dynamics of the family may often be useful in understanding such situations, so may the rather simple notion that study may serve to keep at bay the thoughts about hunger, food and weight, which might otherwise be overwhelming. Such behaviour may be described as an obsession in the broad sense of the term. Occasionally anorexic subjects may display true obsessional tendencies. In psychiatric jargon true obsessions are defined as recurrent intrusive thoughts or impulses which are experienced by the subject as foolish or inappropriate but which are nevertheless continued because to fail to do so would cause tension or would be felt to involve the risk of some unspecified disaster. In anorexia nervosa, repeated and unnecessary checking of weight, or other such neurotic behaviour, may occur, although it is the exception rather than the rule.

It is not surprising that the anorexic subject's relationships with those around her usually change. Her view of herself and her view of the world is different. She is struggling to preserve a precarious position in the face of many pressures. Most of those around her will be trying to get her to eat more normally and to put on weight. For as long as possible she will keep her preoccupations to herself. She is usually unable to understand why she feels as she does, and will almost always be unable to explain her state to others. Those around her may respond with concern, withdrawal, anger, denial, discipline or attempts at producing change by wooing or cajoling. Commonly the reaction is a mixture of all of these, but once the anorexia nervosa is an 'issue' it will often come to be the central and dominating part of the relationship between the subject and anyone who is important to her. Just as with the anorexic's eating behaviour, her relationships may tend to become stuck rigidly in a somewhat distorted pattern or may be erratic and unstable. Interestingly, and perhaps not surprisingly, the patterns of eating and the patterns of interpersonal relationships often run parallel. Thus the abstinent anorexic tends to withdraw into a fixed and often narrow routine of human contact, whereas the overeater may, by contrast, tend towards a more varied pattern of relationships which can come to be both frantic and chaotic.

The sexual feeling and drive of the anorexic subject is invariably reduced but sexual behaviour is by no means always absent. Of course, many subjects, as a consequence of their age, their circumstances or their personality, have had little or no experience of sexual activity. Those who overeat and vomit are more likely to have had sexual intercourse before their illness and to remain sexually active within it (Beumont, George and Smart, 1976). Again, erratic or even promiscuous sexual relationships may be a feature of the general chaos and loss of control which often follows the development of this pattern of eating. Sometimes it seems that such relationships are attempts by the young person to secure hastily some kind of contact with a world which has slipped from her grip. Anorexics rarely report much true sexual feeling or enjoyment in such activity. In a few instances where an abstinent anorexic remains sexually active, she usually seems to be doing so out of a need for security or a sense of obligation or both.

Anorexic subjects show and probably feel rather variable amounts of emotional distress. In the next chapter the idea will be developed that primary anorexia nervosa can be viewed as a way of coping with and avoiding emotional turmoil which might otherwise be or seem to be unmanageable. Thus the degree of distress experienced by the anorexic may be interpreted in part as reflecting its relative success or failure as such a means of coping. Furthermore, the exercise of rigid self-control can be directly rewarding. Hilde Bruch, a leading authority on anorexia nervosa, tells the story of the young Spaniard who prefers to sit in the sun and starve rather than work (Bruch, 1973). When asked about his behaviour he replies that 'in hunger, I am King'. This sense of mastery is not an uncommon feeling among abstinent anorexics, but it is not usually constant or persistent. Anorexia nervosa brings many difficulties and discomforts. Caught between the devil and the deep blue sea, between the fear of weight gain and the reality of illness, a degree of distress is usual, although the subject may often choose to hide it. In general, however, anorexics show depression and anxiety only to a moderate degree (Stonehill and Crisp, 1977). Once again an overeating anorexic who feels quite out of control may become very distressed and may even attempt suicide. Likewise, such subjects may use alcohol or drugs in order to contain their feelings in a way which would be unusual for those whose eating pattern is predominantly an abstinent one.

Anorexic behaviour can be understood as a consequence of the subject's strivings to maintain herself in an abnormal biological position. Her whole way of construing the world and her view of her own body will be coloured by this struggle. Thus although she may seem painfully thin to others the anorexic may perceive her own body as well covered or even as fat and bloated. This misperception of body size can be very striking.

Cynthia was a 20-year-old nursery nurse who had had anorexia nervosa complicated by laxative abuse for three years. She was admitted to a general medical ward for weight restoration when her weight slumped to below 5 stones (32 kg). At this weight she was grossly emaciated. Nevertheless, she would often examine her thighs and abdomen, and then in a childlike voice complain about the fat which she was able to detect beneath her skin. She denied that she was excessively thin. If she was pressed to talk further about the matter, she would hide under the bedclothes and weep.

The way anorexic subjects see their body size was studied more systematically in 1973 by Dr P. D. Slade and Professor G. F. M. Russell. Anorexics were asked to judge when an indicator line was the same width as various parts of their body. In general they overestimated their body size considerably. This study has been repeated and largely confirmed, but it now seems that a tendency to overestimate body size may not be as specific to anorexia nervosa as it was considered to be at one time. It seems that anorexics share this tendency to some degree with the obese, with pregnant women and indeed with a number of non-anorexic young women. It may be that the common factor is a high level of concern about body size and shape (Button, Fransella and Slade, 1977).

The physical features of anorexia nervosa

There is general agreement that certain types of physical disorder are characteristic of anorexia nervosa. Controversy occurs, however, as to whether psychological or physical change is to be thought of as primary, and this will be discussed later. This chapter will describe some of the bodily features and complications of the disorder, although the description and discussion of the major disruptions of hormonal function will in the main be left until Chapter 4. Likewise, the issue of body weight has been and will be covered elsewhere. Weight and hormonal function are the two physical matters which are included in the criteria outlined by Russell. An abnormally low body weight and absent menstrual periods in women are necessary for the diagnosis of anorexia nervosa. Nevertheless, even these apparently simple criteria can be difficult to apply in a few cases. For instance, sometimes those who overeat and vomit may come to be at a fairly normal weight for a while although in other respects they are still in a state which closely resembles anorexia nervosa. When this state persists it clearly presents an affront to strict rules of diagnosis and should not really be described as anorexia nervosa. The term bulimia nervosa is still applicable however. This normal weight eating disorder will be discussed briefly later in this chapter. Likewise, use of the contraceptive pill or other hormonal preparations may cause a kind of menstruation to continue when it would not otherwise do so, and so complicate diagnosis and definition. These, however, are no more than occasional diagnostic traps. What physical features occur regularly apart from low weight and absent menses?

An anorexic subject suffers many discomforts. The rate of her metabolism is turned down as befits a starving creature. Usually her skin is cold. Her arms and legs may be bluish because of the reduction in the volume of blood circulating in them. She may feel cold and at extremes of weight loss, layers of woolly clothing may serve not only to hide her body but also to keep it warm. However, the anorexic who suddenly overeats may undergo a rapid change in metabolic rate and may become flushed and hot. Interesting changes in body hair may represent the remains of primitive biological adaptations to starvation and its attendant problems of heat conservation. Thus many anorexics develop an increase in general body hair. The term 'lanugo' is used to denote this fine silky hair which in a few cases is a remarkable feature of the condition. The hair of the head is also probably increased and certainly diffuse hair loss may occur as an anorexic subject regains weight, particularly if weight restoration occurs rapidly over a few weeks. The hair loss is self-limiting, however, and probably represents the shedding of excess hair which grew in response to undernutrition. While it is easy to speculate that hairiness might have come to be selected as an appropriate response to hard times in the course of evolution, the mechanism and details of hair change in anorexia nervosa remain obscure and they are of little importance clinically.

Symptoms relating to the stomach, gut and bowels (gastrointestinal symptoms) are of more significance for the health of the subject. While such symptoms and difficulties may be important medical indicators, they may also lead to the first contact between the anorexic and those who might be able to help her. Thus, constipation may promote symptoms such as abdominal pain. Not uncommonly an anorexic subject will make tentative appeals for help while concealing the real difficulty, at least at first. Such overtures may provide important clues for the perceptive physician. Occasionally a young woman who is inducing diarrhoea with large doses of purgatives may nevertheless allow herself to be investigated for the symptom. Sometimes there are subjective disorders of swallowing and certainly the complaint of minor abdominal pain and 'indigestion' after eating is common. Rarely the true abdominal emergency of so-called acute dilatation of the stomach occurs.

The physical effects of either laxative abuse or habitual vomiting can be serious. The healthy human body maintains the principal chemical elements of its bodily fluids in careful balance. The concentrations of such ions as sodium and potassium are regulated so as to remain within narrow limits. Each cell contributes to the preservation of the different levels of such substances both inside and outside it. For the body as a whole the hormonal system and the kidneys play crucial roles in this regulation, while the digestive tract is, of course, the site of the absorption of all vital nutrients. However, in abstinent anorexia the intake is reduced and the anorexic denies herself the usual quota of essential elements. Enforced vomiting and, especially, purgative abuse results in an important loss of digestive juices. The economy of the body may suffer increasing depletions, particularly of potassium, and its regulating mechanisms may be put under great strain and even overwhelmed sometimes. The kidney may malfunction when potassium is scarce and a vicious circle is created. Epileptic fits occur in a substantial proportion of anorexic individuals, and mostly happen in the context of deranged internal chemistry. Furthermore, the depletion of potassium in the heart can be fatal. Nevertheless, some chronically depleted subjects do seem to tolerate and survive extraordinary deviations from the normal in a way which probably represents an adaptation of their body systems to their persistently abnormal internal environments. However, their position is always precarious. There is no doubt that the imbalances produced by chronic diarrhoea and vomiting place the individual in a truly dangerous position. Thus the vomiting anorexic runs some risks which the abstaining anorexic avoids, although it is certainly possible to get into serious metabolic problems through abstinence alone.

It is probably true to say that little is known of the detailed mechanism of some of the states of physical disorder which can sometimes be seen in anorexia nervosa. For instance, the boggy swelling (oedema) of the legs which may occur at times is by no means fully understood. However, almost invariably these states recover fully if the weight and feeding behaviour of the subject returns to normal.

Anorexia nervosa in the male

Boys and men do develop primary anorexia nervosa, but they do so much less commonly than girls and young women. Even so, anorexia nervosa in the male may be more common than it seems to be. The disorder may not be considered readily by a doctor when faced with a male patient. It is commonly thought of as a female condition. Indeed, without the cessation of menstruation as a symptom, it is much more difficult for a doctor to be sure of the diagnosis. Nevertheless, in the definite case the subject's low weight, odd eating habits and his attitude to both will be enough to make a clinical diagnosis possible. Investigation can reveal similar patterns of hormonal change to that which underlies the amenorrhoea in the female.

There have been few descriptions of male anorexics in the medical literature. These descriptions tend to agree that in general the behaviour of anorexic men and boys resembles closely that of their female counterparts. However, a few differences have been suggested.

There seems to be some evidence that those males who become anorexic tend to do so on average at an earlier age than females. Likewise, the social class bias may be less evident, with relatively more male anorexics coming from working-class homes. Some authors have suggested that a family history of anorexia nervosa is particularly common in male cases. Finally there is an impression that male anorexics respond to treatment less well and may be more likely to become chronic or to drop out of follow-up treatment. Indeed, it would make sense if those few males who do become anorexic are products of environments in which feelings toward the disorder are particularly strong, as might occur if other family members have the condition; given these major pressures,

male anorexics in this situation might be expected to recover less
easily.

Chronic anorexia nervosa

There is no agreed length of time after which a person is generally
considered to be suffering from chronic anorexia nervosa. Likewise,
there are no absolute features which are characteristic of chronicity.
Nevertheless, the term chronic may be useful to denote, albeit
loosely, a state where the condition has been long-lasting and the
subject seems to be firmly stuck within it. Thus a young woman
who has been anorexic for half-a-dozen years or so will probably
have spent a quarter or more of her life and almost certainly over
half of her time since puberty within the condition. In many ways
her experiences will be widely separated from those of her contemporaries. Such an individual may manage to make something of
her life in spite of her disorder. A kind of encapsulation occurs and
she may separate her life into compartments, in some of which she
may cope quite well. Her working life, for example, may often be
relatively successful. However, characteristically she will have difficulty in personal relationships as well as in the narrow matters of
eating, weight and health. Some women marry while anorexic although owing to their amenorrhoea they are, of course, infertile. In
such a marriage, the anorexic will often choose a partner who suits
her as the kind of person she has come to be within the condition.
For instance, the husband may be ordered, quiet and sexually
undemanding, or alternatively superficially glamorous but privately
wary of personal or sexual involvement. The marriage may be
stable while the wife remains anorexic but will often be strained and
tested if and when a process of recovery begins. Indeed the marriage
may break down altogether unless both partners can adjust to the
important changes which recovery brings.

The lives of some chronic anorexics show less accommodation
and remain dominated by the disorder. As time passes some abstinent anorexics recover while others develop the overeating and
vomiting pattern of behaviour. Vomiters, therefore, form a substantial proportion of chronic anorexics, probably over half. The life-
style of such persons can become quite bizarre.

Rachel was 24 years old and had had anorexia nervosa for eight years. For over five years she had been overeating and vomiting. She had sought help from a number of doctors but had failed to escape from the condition. At times her overeating was gross. Her weight varied widely from quite low to within the normal range and there had been a tendency over recent years for her mean weight to increase. However, her eating disorder remained severe. She lived alone in London and worked in a clerical job which she found boring and undemanding. At the time of presentation, she described her summer evening activity as follows. She would go into the West End of London and wander around the streets or bars where she would try to meet and get into conversation with tourists. She would then offer to show them good places to eat and would go with them to a restaurant and usually be treated to a large meal. As she finished the meal she would make an excuse, leave and then vomit up the food which she had eaten. Sometimes she would then go in search of more tourists, and the process was repeated.

In such cases the apparatus of anorexic behaviour, which at first seemed merely a means by which the subject avoided a normal weight, takes over the person's life. Paradoxically, the subject's preoccupation with eating sometimes may come to override even her concern about weight. However, for the majority weight and eating are inextricably mixed and become the concepts which dominate the world of the chronic anorexic.

Bulimia nervosa

Some anorexic individuals have a body weight in the normal range and yet persist in a disturbed pattern of eating for months or even years. Binge eating comes to dominate the condition, although enforced vomiting or laxative abuse together with a fearful concern about control of weight and eating are also involved. Some arrive at this position without ever having been in a state of primary anorexia nervosa. This condition is described as the bulimic syndrome or as bulimia nervosa, although the latter term is also applied to individuals who have low weight anorexia nervosa with prominent overeating (bulimia). The outlook for sufferers from bulimia nervosa is probably highly variable and for some it is merely a stage on the road to recovery or is just a brief episode. However, there is no doubt that bulimia at normal weight can also become a state which entraps the sufferer no less miserably than does anorexia nervosa. Recently considerable progress has been made in developing specific psychotherapeutic techniques for this disorder (Fairburn, 1981; Lacey, 1983). These usually involve the combination of psychological treatment with dietary advice and monitoring. However, the detailed discussion of bulimic disorder at normal weight is outside the scope of this book (for further information see Palmer, 1987).

Prognosis

It is surprisingly difficult to describe the 'natural history' of untreated anorexia nervosa. It is uncertain how many people in the population have ever been in the condition, just as what happens to those who never come to medical attention and how their anorexic career differs from treated patients is difficult to know. People who observe and report upon series of anorexic subjects are usually doctors or others who are keen to help. Therefore, most of the anorexics who have been described have also been treated in some way. Furthermore, doctors who write about any condition tend to gain a reputation which leads people to seek them out to help with particularly serious or difficult cases. So the anorexics who are described in the medical literature may not be typical of anorexics in treatment who may in turn not be typical of anorexics in general. Current views may underestimate the number of people experiencing the condition but may tend to overestimate its probable seriousness in any one individual.

Death or truly chronic illness may be the outcome of the disorder in perhaps one in ten cases which come to the attention of doctors. As was described above, some people with anorexia nervosa remain ill for long periods, often a decade or more. Their lives are changed and distorted by the disorder in a way from which they may never truly escape. The experience of a time when their life was constrained in this way will necessarily leave a scar upon their subsequent development even if they recover in terms of their weight and eating. Some such subjects undoubtedly emerge eventually into a non-anorexic state, although some may be well into middle age by the time they do so. Others will succumb to the disorder by inanition, metabolic disorder or by suicide. The reported mortality from the disorder in series of anorexic patients has at times been as high as 10 per cent. This is certainly an overestimate of the condition in general, but it is important to emphasize that anorexia nervosa is still a disorder from which people die. In 1975, twelve people between the ages of fifteen and fifty (eleven females and one male) were certified as having died of anorexia nervosa in the United Kingdom. Most, but not all, of these deaths probably arose through true primary anorexia nervosa. At the other extreme perhaps a further 10 per cent or so of anorexics who contact doctors recover quickly after an illness lasting just a few months. However, most identified anorexics, who make up a central group, become stuck within the condition for a period from several months to a few years but often emerge from the disorder in response to treatment.

3 · An attempt at explanation

The last chapter was concerned mainly with description, inasmuch as one can describe a complex state such as primary anorexia nervosa without attempts at explanation intruding. In general, it is probable that most doctors and other professionals who have seen many cases of the disorder would recognize and agree that the picture of it presented in this book fits broadly with their experience, though some might wish to change details or shift the emphasis.

There is a good deal less consensus on the question of the nature of the disorder and how it is to be best understood and explained. One authority may discuss the disorder with an emphasis on the unconscious and symbolic aspects of food and eating, while another authority may seem to be concerned almost exclusively with a discussion of the transmission of information within the brain by small neurotransmitter molecules and their possible significance in feeding disorders. Those involved with the behavioural sciences in general and perhaps psychiatrists and clinical psychologists in particular have of necessity become accustomed to such a bewildering range of discourse. Too often perhaps our preferred way of coping is to shut our eyes and stop our ears to most of the hubbub and quietly attend to our own little patch using well-worn conceptual tools, only occasionally raising our heads to look over the fence to shout encouragement or abuse at the neighbours. To the outsider it must seem a rather odd state of affairs and indeed it is, since there is much to be gained from the critical exchange and combination of these different kinds of understanding. In fact, anorexia nervosa seems to demand such an approach. Certainly the most satisfactory attempts to explain the nature of the disorder are those which combine ideas derived from observations of a widely differing kind. To this end, this chapter is concerned with presenting a way of looking at anorexia nervosa which may serve as a framework around which a variety of observations may be arranged. It must be emphasized that it is only *one* way of looking at the disorder and should not be construed as some final 'truth'.

Entanglement

It may be useful to consider that anorexia nervosa involves the gross and inappropriate entanglement of two issues: on the one hand, weight and eating control, and, on the other, what might be described as personal and emotional control. For either or both of these to be a source of some concern to the individual is not unusual but severe disorders arise when the two sets of issues become malignantly involved.

What is meant by weight and eating control is probably clear but the issue of personal and emotional control may need clarification. Self-esteem and self-evaluation are the pivotal issues while the extent to which a person feels in control of his or her own destiny and emotions comes into play as well. These issues are of concern to everyone to a greater or lesser extent. The anorexic may be thought of as having an average or greater than average lack of confidence but what singles her out is the extent to which these issues become entangled with her weight and eating control. A degree of such entanglement is not unusual in our society. Appearance and body size and shape are issues which may be of considerable importance, particularly to young women, in determining the individual's degree of self-esteem. The anorexic, however, exaggerates the importance of her weight and shape and may develop highly unusual ideas about how they relate to her well-being. More importantly still, she will characteristically feel that her grasp upon these issues is tenuous and that she is always about to lose control. As a result, she feels that if she allows herself to eat a little more than she intends there is a real possibility of losing control of eating altogether; furthermore, if shc allows her weight to rise a little she feels that it will go on rising in a similarly uncontrolled manner. These fantasies about losing control are perhaps central to an understanding of anorexia nervosa. They come about initially through the dilemmas experienced by the individual who seeks to impose excessive restraints on her weight and eating; the response to these dilemmas arises out of and confirms the entanglement of ideas mentioned above. To understand this cycle further it is necessary to outline a way of looking at weight and eating control.

Weight and eating control

The mechanisms involved in the control of human body weight and eating are poorly understood but are undoubtedly complex, involving biological, psychological and social elements. However, in spite of this complexity and uncertainty there is widespread belief in a remarkably simple model of weight and eating control which one might describe as the 'slimming philosophy'. According to this view, body weight is controlled by simple economic laws of input and output; theoretically, it is possible to achieve and maintain any desired weight by manipulating these factors. In addition, it is frequently implied that the manipulation of body weight to a desired level will also produce changes in body shape towards whatever is construed as ideal. The importance society places on presentation is reinforced by the existence of a prosperous industry which espouses such ideas and sells products which claim to help the consumer to put them into practice. It is worthy of note that there is no such industry which claims to help people to change their height since height in adults is generally accepted as something which an individual is stuck with whether they like it or not. While weight is mutable and height is not, it seems likely that the slimming philosophy grossly exaggerates the ease with which body weight and size can be changed and, furthermore, the extent to which this influences body shape. Arguments against this simple view include the remarkable stability of most people's body weight and the typical course of most attempts to change it. It is certainly true that, for whatever reason, the vast majority of attempts to modify body weight by slimming end in failure. A further objectionable aspect of the simple slimming philosophy is that an individual who is dissatisfied with her body weight and seeks to change it but fails not only remains dissatisfied but also must construe herself as having made insufficient effort or having used the wrong technique. Thus her fatness is not only thought of as a misfortune but also as a failing. Such beliefs tend to increase the degree of entanglement between weight and eating control and wider issues of self-esteem.

In contrast to the slimming philosophy there is considerable evidence that human body weight is, in fact, a regulated system. This means that body weight will tend to resist change and stay at a set point. Indeed for most people the evidence is that body weight is remarkably steady most of the time in spite of the lack of detailed attention to calorie input which the simple slimming philosophy would seem to demand. Undoubtedly, changes in body weight do occur over time (for instance, the phenomenon of 'middle-age spread' is real enough) but they tend to occur slowly and are only evident against the background of inherent stability. On the other hand, some people's stable weight changes fairly quickly; the reasons for this, as with many of the phenomena associated with weight control, are largely unknown.

The inherent stability of human body weight does not stop people being dissatisfied with the weight at which they are apparently 'set'. Indeed, it is commonplace for people in our society to want to be at least a few pounds lighter than they find themselves although there are also a few people who see themselves as being unduly skinny and whose aim is to gain weight. The idea of a natural weight regulation would predict that both of these groups would find changing their weight more difficult than they had anticipated, and indeed they do.

What might be called the 'natural history' of an attempt at slimming would seem to be something as follows. An individual decides to try to lower his or her body weight and logically seeks to do so by restraining the urge to eat and by cutting back on the amount of food eaten daily or, in particular, the calorie count of the food consumed. Often this will include the avoidance of foods perceived as especially 'fattening' such as greasy or high-carbohydrate foods. Typically, this enterprise goes well at first and is associated with positive feelings of determination, resolve, self-control and accomplishment as the first few pounds are lost. Sooner or later, however, these positive accompaniments of slimming will come to be challenged by more negative consequences of self-imposed dietary restraint. These include hunger, preoccupation with food, a sensitivity to external cues for eating, a tendency towards bingeing if control is relaxed and, lastly, a generally heightened emotional state.

These negative consequences of dietary restraint tend to push the slimmer towards eating more and regaining the lost weight. Whatever the nature of the regulatory mechanisms involved they are forced into a position whereby they push in one direction with increased force as the deviation from their original set point widens. Whereas to the person who is at a 'normal' weight the mechanisms are little evident and 'friendly', to the slimmer they become increasingly an 'unfriendly' force opposing the intention of the diet. Instead of being a source of gentle regulatory control the mechanisms take on the nature of a potentially disruptive jack-in-the-box. Characteristically the typical would-be slimmer gives up the struggle in the face of these forces and most slimming diets end up in 'failure' and an eventual restoration of something like the original weight. It can be argued that such a response is usually the most healthy and sensible one; however, it is not the response of the person who is about to develop anorexia nervosa.

The anorexic response

The previous section outlined what might be called the dieter's dilemma. The dilemma arises from the fact that an attempt at slimming does not consist of a simple move from one stable position to another as would be predicted by the slimming philosophy. Rather, it is characterized by a move from a position of stability to one of instability and increasing pressure to return to the status quo. Change can be achieved but usually only at the expense of experiencing the negative consequences of eating restraint. This price is too high for most people; the matter is simply insufficiently important to them. For the anorexic-to-be, the enterprise of slimming is perhaps already greatly entangled with wider issues of self-esteem and seems to be of more importance. Furthermore, the consequences of letting go and giving up seem frightening. As a result her response to the aversive consequences of slimming is different and she battles against them. Her hunger may in part be denied, while the word 'hunger' itself may be thought to be 'homely' and, as such, inapplicable. She will say that she experiences an urge to eat, in spite of the fact that she is 'not hungry'. She will be preoccupied with food and eating but the preoccupation may be channelled into food theory, cooking for others or ritualizing the preparation and eating of what she does allow herself. She will find herself sensitive to external cues for eating but will seek to manage her life so as to avoid these. The impulse to binge may be present but will be fought against as an evil self-indulgence which must be defeated, a view that is fostered rather than refuted if she does succumb. Lastly, the heightened emotional state of the semi-starved person serves to confirm the sense of entanglement between control of eating and wider emotional issues and hints at what might happen if she did indeed let herself go. Her fantasy is of total loss of control.

Faced with this fear and this fantasy the anorexic-to-be postpones the risky business of letting go and giving up and opts instead for continued restraint. Unfortunately, motivated as it is by fear of the consequences of the forces promoted by restraint, this response results in the creation of a vicious circle; the more she persists in restraint, the greater these forces become and the greater the sense of risk involved in escaping. She is trapped. What is more, the longer she continues, the more important the battle for her general well-being and self-esteem becomes. Yet, as with any vicious circle, it is a battle that cannot be won. Her shaky self-esteem is dependent upon a vicious and hopeless struggle and is further undermined.

Entrapment

Most individuals who suffer from anorexia nervosa will have followed this career. As has been emphasized above, a few individuals reach a similar position in which a low body weight is combined with an unimpaired appetite for some reason other than self-imposed slimming. Whatever the reason, there may well be many factors in common, especially concerning the development of an entanglement between issues of weight and eating control and the wider issues which have already been discussed. This entanglement can go on to include the development of the increasingly firmly held but sometimes bizarre ideas which characterize the thinking of the established sufferer. Furthermore, the established disorder brings with it unsettling consequences for the anorexic and her relationship with others, which may in turn increase the degree of entrapment.

The state of nutritional deprivation in which the anorexic now finds herself has physical consequences, especially for her hormonal status. In many ways these changes closely resemble a retreat from biological adulthood to a state that was normal before puberty. To an individual struggling with personal difficulties which may be thought of as aspects of the continuing process of growing up, such a retreat may in some sense be a relief. These biological factors may contribute to the trap and will be discussed at greater length in the next chapter.

4 · *Hormones, the brain and anorexia nervosa*

Hormonal messages are of great importance in the control system of the human body. Hormones are secreted in tiny quantities by the specialized tissues of the endocrine glands. The term *endocrine* denotes that the secretions of these glands pass into the bloodstream, in contrast to the *exocrine* glands which pass their secretions, usually in much larger quantities, into the gut or on to the body surface. (The sweat glands and salivary glands are examples of exocrine glands. The thyroid and the adrenals are examples of endocrine glands.) Hormones, rather like drugs, have effects upon bodily function and metabolism which seem quite out of proportion to the minute amount of their substance. For example, the hormones secreted by the thyroid gland in the neck play an important role in regulating the general rate of body metabolism and yet the relevant hormones are present in the body fluids in concentrations which are measured in micrograms. The number of hormones and hormone-like substances which have been described is large and still growing.

The centre of control and responsiveness in the body is, of course, the nervous system and especially the brain. The nervous system and the endocrine system are closely linked and work together. The endocrine system tends to be organized as an array of tiers with the pituitary gland (or hypophysis) acting as a link between the brain and the more distant endocrine glands for several functions. For a generation of medical students the pituitary was invariably described as 'the conductor of the endocrine orchestra'. Although hackneyed, the phrase was apt since this small gland, positioned in a bony compartment in the middle of the skull, secretes hormones which regulate the endocrine functions of the adrenal cortex, the thyroid and the sex organs (gonads) in both sexes. The pituitary gland is really two structures which have come together in the course of development. The posterior pituitary (or neurohypophysis) is essentially a part of the brain and is concerned with the secretion of hormones which play a part in the regulation of the kidneys and probably also in childbirth and lactation. The anterior pituitary (or adenohypophysis) is derived from a piece of tissue from the gut which moves as the embryo develops until it comes to lie against the posterior pituitary to form one structure which remains, however, in these two distinct parts. The anterior pituitary is concerned with the release of at least six hormones, four of which have their effects by controlling the actions of other endocrine glands situated elsewhere in the body. The release of the pituitary hormones is controlled in turn by a set of about seven hormones (sometimes called releasing factors) which are produced within an adjacent part of the brain known as the hypothalamus. These hypothalamic hormones pass from the brain to the anterior pituitary along a special system of small blood-vessels known as the hypophysial portal system. Thus the brain and the endocrine glands are intimately linked together and the links between the hypothalamus and the pituitary are such as to make it more sensible to talk in terms of a *neuroendocrine* system. The parts of this neuroendocrine system influence each other by being variably responsive to the circulating levels of the hormones. Feedback loops, both negative and positive, contribute to a complex control system, which is, however, subject to the overriding influence of the brain. The brain is, of course, sensitive to both the internal and external environments of the body, but is influenced by the hormones in the blood and the fluids which bathe it. It is mainly through the brain, however, that external environmental influences have their effects upon the neuroendocrine system and hence upon the functions which it regulates.

An example may clarify the tiered nature of the neuroendocrine system. The sex hormone system in the female may be especially relevant to anorexia nervosa, although the broad pattern applies to the male sex hormone system and to other systems in both sexes. Many aspects of bodily structure and functions in the adult human female are influenced by the circulating levels of the hormones produced in the ovaries. The menstrual cycle is perhaps the clearest example of a change which is largely controlled by the prevailing mix of ovarian hormones. There are two main types of *ovarian hormone*, oestrogen and progesterone. (In fact, each type is represented by more than one active substance, and the ovary also produces some androgens, 'male' sex hormones.) These two main types of ovarian hormone are made in differing amounts at different times, and their relative levels control the changes in the lining of the uterus which at the end of the cycle results in menstrual loss. The varying levels of the ovarian hormones are the result of changes of structure and function which are going on in the ovary where the ovum ('egg') is developed and then ejected (ovulation), if unfertilized, by a tiny cluster of cells called the follicle. A new follicle is developed each month and, after the ovum is ejected, it changes its form and becomes known as a corpus luteum. The biological function of the process is, of course, to develop an ovum and prepare the uterus for its reception and further growth should it become fertilized.

Thus, the cyclical changes in the uterus are controlled by the changes in the proportions and concentrations of oestrogen and progesterone in the blood reaching it, which in turn are the result of the changes going on in the ovary. The ovarian changes are subject to the control of hormones from the anterior pituitary gland. These hormones are known collectively as *gonadotrophins* because they influence the gonads (sex organs, i.e., ovaries or testes). There are two gonadotrophins. They are known as the follicular stimulating hormone (FSH) and luteinizing hormone (LH) because their major influence seems to be upon the follicle and the corpus luteum respectively. The relative concentrations of FSH and LH control the ovarian changes, but further up the system the release of these gonadotrophins from the pituitary is controlled by a hypothalamic hormone secreted into the portal blood supply from the brain. There seems to be only one hypothalamic hormone involved in the control of both gonadotrophins. It has been known by several names, including the cumbersome luteinizing hormone releasing hormone, or, worse, luteinizing hormone/follicular stimulating hormone releasing hormone, but perhaps its most satisfactory name is gonadotrophin releasing hormone or GRH for short. Precisely how this single releasing hormone can promote the independent secretion of both FSH and LH is unclear at present, although it would be a fair guess to suggest that the already prevailing levels of the pituitary and

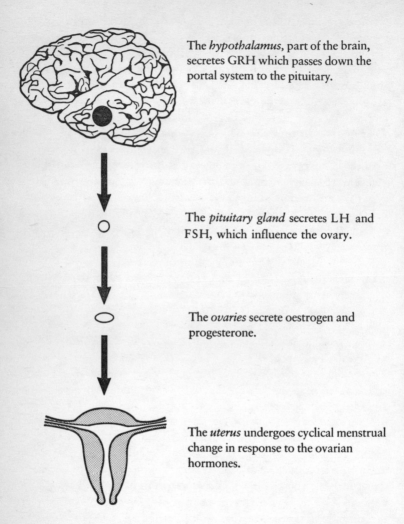

The *hypothalamus*, part of the brain, secretes GRH which passes down the portal system to the pituitary.

The *pituitary gland* secretes LH and FSH, which influence the ovary.

The *ovaries* secrete oestrogen and progesterone.

The *uterus* undergoes cyclical menstrual change in response to the ovarian hormones.

The diagram indicates a flow of information and control from the hypothalamus to the uterus. However, the hypothalamus is undoubtedly influenced by other parts of the brain and by circulating hormones.

Fig. 1   Schematic representation of the tiered control of the menstrual cycle

ovarian hormones play an important part in determining the response of the pituitary to the arrival of GRH from the hypothalamus. The brain, the anterior pituitary and the ovaries thus contribute to a three-tiered system which influences the uterus, the so-called target organ (see Fig. 1). The complexity of the system presumably allows a combination of sensitivity with smooth control.

The brain and endocrine glands as a whole form a system which has important and widespread effects upon the body and its functions. It is important to note, however, that the peripheral endocrine glands and indeed their target organs influence the brain in turn. There is feedback from the periphery of both a hormonal and neural kind. Furthermore, it is probably true that even the hypothalamic hormones have direct effects on the brain. Indeed, the brain is probably an important direct target organ of hormonal activity in a way which has been insufficiently emphasized or studied in the past. Anything which influences the brain can influence behaviour.

Neuroendocrine status and behaviour

The neuroendocrine system is undoubtedly involved in our emotional experience and behaviour. Clearly the brain is the seat of our consciousness and there is evidence that the levels of different hormones circulating in the blood may at times show some relationship to the way we feel and act. The hypothalamus in particular seems to play some part in rather basic matters such as appetite and eating, sexual function, aggression and mood. In animals, experimental manipulation of neuroendocrine mechanisms can be shown to result in changes of behaviour. Conversely, changes in the animals' environment can promote changes in neuroendocrine status. However, what is demonstrable in creatures such as the laboratory rat may not be so demonstrable in the human being, for at least two reasons. Firstly, the kind of control and experimental manipulation which is required can rarely be justified ethically for work with human subjects. Thus observations of people tend to be less tightly controlled, or result from chance 'experiments of nature', or are made on highly selected and unrepresentative individuals, or sometimes all three! There would, therefore, be practical difficulties in demonstrating any close parallels between neuroendocrine status and behaviour, should these exist. Secondly, there are reasons to suppose that such links may not be nearly so close in the human. Man's experience and behaviour clearly contain an important dimension which is absent in the laboratory rat and which is understandable only in personal and cultural terms. This dimension must be considered if we are to feel we understand why a fellow human being is behaving in a certain way. As the old adage says, 'One man's meat is another man's poison'. Indeed, perhaps this is particularly appropriate when thinking about anorexia nervosa. We would, therefore, be foolish if ever we felt that our understanding of an individual's behaviour was more than sketchy and provisional. Nevertheless, we should not abandon the notion that the neuroendocrine system is relevant to human experience. To do so would surely be to throw the baby out with the bath water.

When disease of a gland distorts the secretion of a hormone, the functions which the gland would normally regulate will be affected. It is not infrequent in such cases for the emotional state and behaviour of the person to be changed as a consequence of the endocrine disease, although often the changes will stop short of mental illness. For instance, both over- and under-secretion of the thyroid gland (hypo- and hyperthyroidism) can produce psychological changes which may be severe. In hyperthyroidism (often known as thyrotoxicosis) the individual may be very jumpy and anxious, whereas in hypothyroidism (myxoedema) the reverse occurs and the subject is tired, slowed down and lethargic. In extreme cases of both disorders true psychosis may occur.

Less marked changes in the levels of various hormones may be detectable after a person has been subjected to experiences which induce emotional states such as fear or sexual arousal. These changes may be short-lived, as in the case of the burst of adrenalin which accompanies fright or excitement, but more prolonged changes of secretion of some hormones may occur also as a response to environmental events. For instance, the increased secretion of the steroid hormones of the adrenal cortex tends to be part of the body's response to more lasting stress.

Thus, even in the human, hormones influence experience and

behaviour, but, conversely, experience and behaviour can influence hormonal levels and the neuroendocrine system in general. It is possible to play philosophical conkers about the nature of such influences, but in practice it is perhaps enough to accept that the relationship between bodily events and behavioural events is an intimate one.

Weight, body fat and puberty

As children grow up they pass through a transition towards physical adulthood known as puberty. In boys the process involves the familiar changes in bulk, in voice and in body hair. Likewise, girls change their shape, begin to develop breasts and so on. These changes take place over many months. In both personal and cultural terms the onset of menstruation (the menarche) tends to be accorded a central significance as a marker of puberty in girls. In scientific and clinical work, too, the menarche is a useful reference point since it can usually be dated with some precision. However, in considering puberty and an individual's neuroendocrine status, it is important to remember that menstruation is used merely as an indicator. Both external and internal changes occur before the menarche and continue after it.

Recent studies would seem to indicate that body weight is a better predictor of the menarche than age or height; better indeed than any other easily measured variable that has been studied (Frisch and Revelle, 1970). At least for European and white American females, a number of crucial developmental milestones seem to be closely linked to the time of attaining certain body weights. The timing of the adolescent growth spurt, of the period of maximum growth rate and of the onset of menstruation all seem to occur at particular weights rather than at particular ages. In the case of the menarche, this weight is around 7 st. 4 lb (47 kg). Clearly there are individual variations and exceptions, since some women attain full sexual maturity and reproductive capacity without ever reaching this weight. Also, it seems likely that different racial groups may well have different average critical weights in this respect; pygmy peoples would be the extreme case. However, for given populations, the menarche is remarkably predictable by means of body weight.

An even better predictor of menarche may be total body fat, although this is more difficult to measure than body weight. However, methods are available by which body fat can be estimated. Much of the investigation of the relationship of weight and body fat with puberty and menstruation has been carried out by Dr Rose Frisch and her colleagues at the Harvard Center for Population Studies in the United States. She speculates that the biological function of the amount of fat which maturing girls seem to require firstly to start menstruating and subsequently to achieve full fertility is concerned with the need to be able to survive a pregnancy even in times of scarcity. Thus she observes that the 2 st. 7 lb (16 kg) of fat which is typical of an 18-year-old girl could, if necessary, provide 144,000 calories and sustain her for the duration of a pregnancy and three months' lactation. It would certainly make sense in evolutionary terms if women became fertile only when they possessed such a fatty insurance policy against hard times.

Such ideas are, of course, speculative. However, it does appear to be an established observation that for populations of broadly similar young women, there is a link between average weight or body fat and the average timing of the menarche. Such averages represent the summation of individual values for weight, body fat and age at menarche. Thus, although the majority of individuals will, for instance, start to menstruate at a weight remarkably close to the mean value for the population from which they are drawn, a few will deviate markedly from this mean. However, it is probable that for each individual there is a close link between a particular body weight or amount of body fat and the onset of puberty. The existence of such a critical weight could only be detected if puberty was reversible, when the critical weight could be passed more than once. Such a reversal may occur when a young person develops anorexia nervosa.

Neuroendocrine changes in anorexia nervosa

The fact that anorexia nervosa leads invariably to the stopping of the menstrual cycle in the female has meant that the endocrine status of individuals suffering from the disorder has always been a subject of interest and study. Indeed, as was mentioned earlier, for the first two or three decades of this century there was considerable confusion and controversy about the relationship between the disorder and primary failure of the pituitary gland (Simmonds' disease). While the distinction between these two conditions has been clear for many years, the clarification of the endocrine states which occur within primary anorexia nervosa has progressed piecemeal as both ideas and techniques of investigation have developed in endocrinology in general. The process continues and there is much that remains unclear. However, it is quite striking that most of the observations of subjects with anorexia nervosa resemble closely those that may be made on much younger subjects who have yet to pass through puberty. Thus the endocrine status of a 19-year-old anorexic will more closely match that of a healthy 9-year-old girl than that of her normal-weight contemporaries.

The lack of periods, of course, immediately suggests a lack of cyclical change in the controlling ovarian hormones, oestrogen and progesterone. Some of the first studies of the hormonal condition of anorexics showed that levels of these hormones excreted in the urine were unusually low and lacked the expected cyclical changes. These observations have now been confirmed with direct measurement of the levels of these hormones in the blood. Furthermore, now that blood levels of the gonadotrophins, FSH and LH, can be measured readily, it has been demonstrated repeatedly that the secretion of these hormones is also markedly reduced in anorexics when they are at a low weight. For instance, in a normal young woman the level of LH in the blood plasma would tend to be of the order of ten or more international units per litre and vary cyclically with a peak at the time of ovulation; in the underweight anorexic the level of LH is usually less than 2 IU/litre and no peaking occurs. Similar observations have been made for the other gonadotrophin, FSH, although the reduction of this hormone often seems to be less marked than that of LH.

Thus the basis of the clinically observed amenorrhoea can be traced back along the control system, firstly to the ovary and its hormones, and then to the pituitary gland and its gonadotrophins. What of the hypothalamic hormone (GRH) which in turn regulates the secretion of the gonadotrophins? It is not possible to measure directly the rate of secretion of GRH. After its release from the hypothalamus it passes down the portal blood-vessels to the

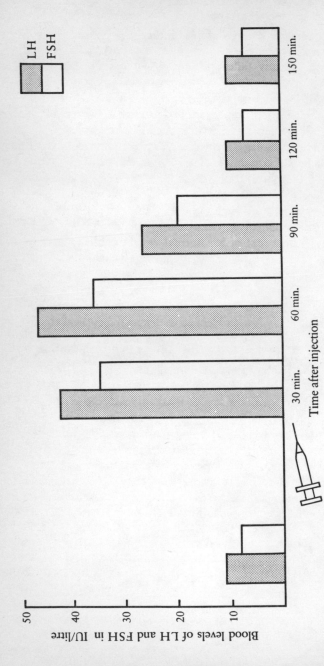

Fig. 2   Typical healthy adult response to the intravenous injection of 50 μg of GRH – a sharp rise in gonadotrophin levels

pituitary and a little probably escapes into the general circulation. However, GRH can be injected and used as a test of the responsiveness of the pituitary, which may reflect the level of 'priming' by endogenous GRH.

When small doses of GRH are injected into the veins of normal young people the response of the pituitary is to increase the release of both FSH and LH for a short time, which is reflected in a transient rise in levels of these hormones in the blood (see Fig. 2). A rise in hormone levels is detectable in samples taken only five minutes after the injection of GRH. The highest levels are usually detectable half to one hour after injection and by two hours the levels of FSH and LH characteristically fall back towards the pre-injection values. The rise in LH levels is normally greater than the corresponding rise in FSH levels.

However, when similar small doses of GRH are given intra-venously to subjects with primary anorexia nervosa who are markedly underweight the response is quite different (see Fig. 3). The increases of FSH and LH tend to be much smaller, giving rise to a flatter response curve, and the rise of LH is usually relatively more flattened than that of FSH. Indeed, if the body weight of the anorexic subject is below about 6½–7 stones (40–45 kg), depending on height, and the dose of GRH is 50 μg or less, the response may be barely detectable (Palmer *et al.*, 1975).

Thus it would seem that at low weights the responsiveness of the pituitary is reduced or even 'switched off'. Does this then reflect primary pituitary disease? This seems unlikely because of the results of simple refeeding without other physical intervention. If an anorexic individual weighing 6 st. 4 lb (40 kg), and with a flattened gonadotrophin response to GRH, gains weight to 7 st. 12 lb (50 kg) the responsiveness of her pituitary will be restored to normal. Indeed as her weight rises her responsiveness may for a time be somewhat greater than average. There is a clear relationship between body weight and the results of the GRH test. Figure 4 shows the increasing response to 50 μg of GRH in a 20-year-old anorexic girl undergoing treatment by means of bed rest, normal mixed diet and psychotherapy. As her weight rises, so does the FSH and LH response. Also, her initially greater FSH response is overtaken by the LH response, and the normal balance of response is restored. Unfortunately,

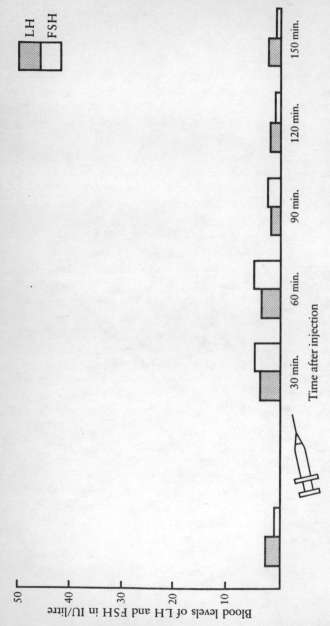

Fig. 3   Gonadotrophin response to the intravenous injection of 50 μg of GRH in an anorexic subject at low weight

she relapsed subsequently and when her weight fell again so did her response to GRH.

The probable interpretation of these findings is that the gona-dotrophin response of the pituitary depends upon the general 'prim-ing' which it has received over time from the person's endogenous GRH coming down from the hypothalamus. These results would indicate that it is the secretion of GRH from the hypothalamus that is, in fact, switched off at low weights. Support for this view comes from the effects of giving repeated high doses of GRH to anorexic women. Doses of 500 μg given three times per day for four weeks have resulted in a restoration of responsiveness and indeed of ovulation and menstruation (Nillius, Fries and Wide, 1975). The mechanism of the disorder is thus traced back into the brain.

There would seem to be a weight-sensitive mechanism in the brain which produces a chain of measurable effects in the neuro-endocrine system as body weight falls to below about 6½–7 stones (40–45 kg), depending on the height of the subject. At this point, the part of the system which involves the reproductive organs is more or less 'switched off'. In this 'switched off' state the levels of ovarian hormones, the levels of gonadotrophins and the response of the pituitary to stimulation come to resemble closely those which would be expected in a child before puberty. Just as the reaching of a critical weight was involved in triggering the changes of puberty, so the fall of body weight seems to lead to a reversal of some of the changes of puberty. The anorexic individual seems to have reverted to a quasi-prepubertal state. Weight is at the centre of her preoc-cupations and weight would also seem to be the key to the neuro-endocrine changes.

The nature of the weight-sensitive mechanism in the brain re-mains unknown. Clearly the anorexic state has characteristics other than low weight, but it does seem that most of the neuroendocrine changes parallel body weight more closely than, for instance, diet, length of illness, or degree of overt emotional disturbance. How-ever, it is true that not all anorexic subjects regain normal endo-crine and menstrual function as soon as their weight is back to normal. Often there is a considerable delay, perhaps of months, and it may be that other factors are important here. Clearly, weight and diet are closely linked, but some recovering anorexics continue to eat in an unusual or chaotic way while retaining their weight

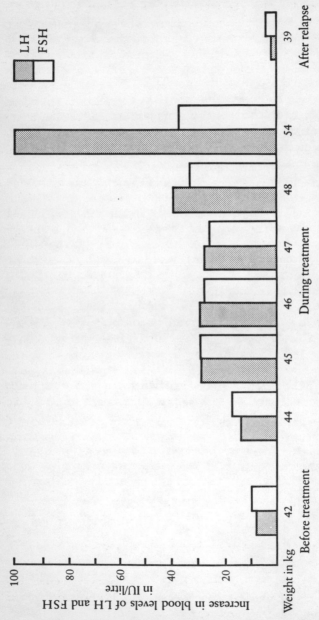

Fig. 4 Maximum observed responses of LH and FSH levels following the intravenous injection of 50 μg of GRH in a 20-year-old anorexic girl as she regains weight, reaches the target weight of 54 kg and then relapses

within normal limits. The response to testing with GRH seems, however, to be almost always recovered when a satisfactory body weight is restored. Likewise, the menstrual cycle seems more able to be restarted by drugs such as clomiphene once the subject is no longer emaciated. Clomiphene interferes with the negative feedback which normally allows the level of ovarian oestrogen to influence the hypothalamus. At low weights, the hypothalamus seems to be resistant to such a 'kick-start' but at higher weights the drug may often restore menstruation (Wakeling *et al.*, 1976). In general, however, if both weight and diet are restored to normal, an anorexic girl may confidently expect her periods to start again within a year at most. Artificial triggering of menstruation is usually neither necessary nor desirable in the treatment of anorexia nervosa.

Endocrine changes in anorexia nervosa are probably not confined to GRH, FSH, LH and the ovarian hormones. The level of the 'male' sex hormone testosterone, which is present in both sexes, tends also to be decreased at low weights and restored with weight gain. The evidence for abnormalities of other hormones is less consistent and impressive. For instance, the secretion of another pituitary hormone known as the growth hormone (GH) probably tends to increase when the anorexic is at a low weight and not eating properly; however, both weight gain and a more normal diet tend to restore normal levels of GH. This hormone has a role in the regulation of body metabolism, particularly that of proteins, and it is probable that the various changes reported in anorexia nervosa reflect the changes in the body's metabolic economy in the face of an erratic diet (Brown *et al.*, 1977). The same may be true of the various observations of changes in thyroid hormones, adrenal cortical hormones and insulin in the condition (Burman *et al.*, 1977; Garfinkel, Brown and Stancer, 1975).

Interpreting the neuroendocrine changes associated with anorexia nervosa

There would seem to be, then, considerable neuroendocrine disorder in anorexic subjects when they are at a low weight. How is this disorder to be best understood?

In general it would seem likely that the disorder of neuroendocrine function is secondary to the changes of nutrition and weight brought about by altered feeding. As we saw above, weight and neuroendocrine function seem to be intimately linked in the initiation of puberty, and the changes which occur with weight loss and anorexia nervosa resemble a reversal of this process. However, there is evidence that suggests that other factors may play a part. For instance, in many series a number of anorexic subjects seem to stop menstruating *before* their weight has fallen below normal or even before they have changed their diet. Furthermore, a very few children seem to develop the disorder before they show any evidence of physical puberty. There are serious objections to the idea that nutritional forces alone determine amenorrhoea and hormonal changes, although it is possible to provide some defence. For instance, finding out the timing of the onset of dieting behaviour is often difficult, especially when the anorexic subject is less than fully frank in telling her story. Some of the reports may, therefore, simply be mistaken. Furthermore, some previously obese subjects could be 'switched off' at a weight which is actually above the average for their height and age, because they are somehow 'set' at this higher level. Such an idea is speculative, although there is some evidence that those subjects whose hormones recover only slowly after weight restoration are those who have been quite fat before their illness (Crisp *et al.*, 1973). Also, in some cases, although the periods may stop, the neuroendocrine disorder may not be the typically profound one of anorexia nervosa until weight loss ensues. Young girls often miss periods for reasons which are either unknown or construed as emotional. Such missed periods may indicate just the kind of vulnerability which makes the subject a candidate for anorexia nervosa. Thus, amenorrhoea as such may be a poor indicator of endocrine status. Likewise, in those rare cases when girls fall ill with anorexia nervosa before there is external evidence of physical puberty it may be that the neuroendocrine changes of puberty began before the disorder cut them short. All in all it seems likely that semi-starvation and weight loss are the most important factors in promoting the endocrine change. These changes are therefore largely an effect of the self-imposed dietary restraint and are initiated by the person in ways that can be best understood in psychological terms. However, it does seem probable that these changes in turn have psychological effects.

People who develop anorexia nervosa are, with very few exceptions, either prepubescent or, more commonly, have gone through puberty in recent years; hence it can be viewed as a disorder of adolescence. Adolescence may be described as the process of change and adjustment in the individual and his or her approach to relationships demanded by growing up and, in particular, by the biological changes of puberty. While puberty is a weight-related event, it would seem that weight loss and semi-starvation can bring a kind of retreat into a quasi pre-pubertal state in which many of the biological effects of adolescence are, as it were, 'switched off'. It would seem entirely plausible that such a retreat might bring psychological changes which were relieving to an individual who was having trouble negotiating adolescence. For the adolescent who is not in difficulty any biological changes which accompany weight loss are less likely to be rewarding. Once established in a 'switched off' position the vulnerable individual may become frightened of weight gain because of its implications of 'switching on' again. The degree of entanglement between weight and eating control and wider personal issues is thereby increased and once again the process of entrapment becomes more secure. A process of psychobiological regression has taken place which provides the individual with a maladaptive 'solution' to some of her difficulties.

At the other extreme from this regression hypothesis is the school that sees all the manifestations of anorexia nervosa as the products of a primary disease of the neuroendocrine system, notably of the hypothalamus and related areas of the brain. Certainly appetite, satiation, sexuality and emotion are changed in anorexia nervosa and the hypothalamus is involved in the control of them all. Might not the psychological changes which appear to promote the disorder, in fact, simply be the result of disease in this part of the brain? It seems unlikely. Firstly, there seems to be no consistent evidence of structural disorder in the brain of anorexic subjects, although it is true that very rarely people with tumours or other lesions in the centre of their brains do develop a state which resembles anorexia nervosa. Secondly, in the majority of cases of anorexia nervosa the evidence of functional change of the neuroendocrine system can be completely reversed by refeeding. Those who seek to explain the whole state as the direct result of brain disease must bear the onus of proof, and so far they have not succeeded in demonstrating any lesion which would support their case.

5 · Psychological and emotional aspects

Anorexia nervosa presents something of a paradox. Young people enter it usually through slimming behaviour which is more or less appropriate. Such slimming may seem to be of a commonplace and unremarkable kind. Furthermore, it is entered into decisively and continued voluntarily. Yet the person who is becoming anorexic is soon distinguished by at least two features. Firstly, she is able to sustain her diet so that she successfully loses weight and, secondly, she comes to feel that her ability to do anything other than continue is diminished. It is as if a trap has closed behind her; she can only remain where she is or push on further in the same direction. How is this state of entrapment to be understood? The last chapter suggested that biological factors may play some part in the development of anorexia nervosa in an individual. This chapter will discuss some of the possible psychological and social factors which may contribute by ensuring the entanglement of self-esteem with the control of weight and eating, thereby making the individual more vulnerable. In general, psychological explanations are probably more convincing at present but the contribution of both biological and social understanding may be crucial as well. Unfortunately, no one simple explanation for the disorder is satisfactory and we are stuck with the view that anorexia nervosa is complex and multi-dimensional. Perhaps in the future some breakthrough will lead to a major simplification and will advance our understanding radically.

It is not difficult to think of possible emotional and psychological influences which could contribute to the disorder. Speculation in psychology is easy and attempts at explanation can sometimes proceed far from the solid ground of evidence and ordered observation. This is fine where such observation and testing follows. Not uncommonly, however, it is difficult to tease out theory from observation and from the necessary informed hunches of clinical practice. Most of what follows in this chapter should be seen as having the status of informally summarized clinical experience and observation, together with informed explanatory speculation. The discussion will be divided somewhat artificially into parts dealing with entry into the disorder and how the disorder may be sustained once established.

Factors which may contribute to the initiation of anorexia nervosa

Many people try to lose weight. Some because of concern about their health; others because they wish to change their appearance. To be slim is widely held to be a sign of relative fitness and there is some evidence to support this view. Likewise, the majority opinion in Western societies at present is that to be slim increases a person's chances of being considered attractive or even beautiful. This applies especially to young women. Individuals who develop anorexia nervosa by way of slimming, diet to lose weight with considerable force and determination. It could be that they share the motivations of those who do not go on to develop the condition, but experience them with greater force. On the other hand, other factors might be required to explain their more extreme behaviour. However, it may be appropriate first to look at health and appearance as areas which provide initial motivation for the anorexic slimmer.

The concepts of health and fitness certainly crop up commonly in the conversation of many anorexic subjects. Some will eat only those items which are obtained from 'health food' shops. Fatty foods are often described as being unhealthy or 'bad'. It is not uncommon for an anorexic subject to adopt a vegetarian diet and give similar explanations for this choice. Sometimes quite bizarre diets may be explained in terms of theories of healthy nutrition which may or may not be cranky but which are sampled and distorted by the anorexic in such a way as to lend support to her own eccentric eating behaviour. At the same time she may be keen on exercising more than the average person. Again she may talk about this in terms of wishing to be physically fit. These ideas about fitness and health may be shared by her family. Indeed, it seems that in many such families these matters are held to have exceptional importance and are pursued with great vigour by some or all of the family members. It is not difficult to see how such views might provide powerful motivation for losing weight. However, the anorexic's preoccupation with health and fitness will appear odd and inconsistent when she is clearly making herself unhealthy and unfit. Nevertheless, the inconsistency which is present in the established case may not have been present at the start when she may well have been indeed both overweight and flabby. The continuation of the preoccupation to the point where it becomes so apparently foolish may reflect the strength of this over-valued notion. Alternatively it may represent the preservation of an idea which was formerly of value in an attempt by the bewildered individual to make sense of the experience which she is undergoing. It is a frightening experience to feel changed by nameless forces. Clinging on to familiar concepts such as the pursuit of health and fitness may help the anorexic to explain her own behaviour. Thus, when anorexia nervosa is established such a preoccupation could become a kind of secondary rationalization even though it was a real and important motivation in the beginning.

The same might be true of slimming with the aim of improving the appearance and increasing attractiveness. The anorexic who appears distressingly emaciated and yet protests that to put on any weight would make her unattractive may simply be repeating outworn phrases because she is otherwise quite unable to understand her own fear of the thought of gaining weight. Her ideas may seem quite inappropriate, but they will at least be familiar and comprehensible to those around her. It could be a mistake, however, to accept them as her 'real' motivation, although it must be said that, in general, motivation is a murky area in which certainty is always difficult to pin-point. However, current views of what an attractive female body should look like must surely provide important reasons for slimming in the first place. Many anorexics are overtly fashion conscious and may come from families or peer groups who are also very concerned about appearance. Often the anorexic and her mother have a common interest in such matters, but for both attractiveness is an emotionally overloaded topic. A not uncommon pattern is for the anorexic daughter to be in a state of more or less explicit rivalry with her mother, who may be very concerned with maintaining her own good looks and youthful figure as she progresses through middle age. At times the rivalry may include a covert competition for the attention of the father or even overt competition for another man. Another pattern occurs when the mother is aware of her own lost youth but seeks to live vicariously through her daughter, perhaps by pushing her towards a 'glamorous' career or life-style. Clearly such a relationship provides both the initial motivation, the model and the ways of thinking about herself which could well make a daughter enter into slimming with much more than usual vigour. Furthermore, the mother may remain receptive to her daughter's explanations of her behaviour in terms of the pursuit of physical attractiveness beyond the point when a less involved observer might judge them to be inappropriate.

In discussing the initiation of anorexia nervosa it is important not to neglect the small group of subjects who do not enter the condition by way of slimming. Some lose weight at first through other causes such as physical illness. Then the anorexic may talk about her state using the language of symptoms and disease. Again, as with health and attractiveness, this way of talking about her condition could be simply an attempt at rationalization.

Health, fitness and attractiveness are all concepts about which there is a measure of consensus. In general, people try to lose weight in order to change themselves for the better. Sometimes the expectations of change are more generalized than is appropriate. To be slim comes to seem not only to be marginally more healthy or marginally more attractive, but rather to approach some never quite to be obtained ideal of health and beauty. For women in particular the world of publicity and advertising promotes the ideal of the glamorous which is just beyond the reach of the individual. John Berger, the critic and novelist (1972), has discussed the way women view themselves in our society as follows.

> According to usage and conventions which are at last being ques-
> tioned but have by no means been overcome, the social presence of
> a woman is different in kind from that of a man. A man's presence

is dependent upon the promise of power which he embodies ... By contrast, a woman's presence expresses her own attitude to herself and defines what can and cannot be done to her ... A woman must continually watch herself. She is almost continually accompanied by her own image of herself. Whilst she is walking across a room or whilst she is weeping at the death of her father, she can scarcely avoid envisaging herself walking or weeping. From earliest childhood she has been taught and persuaded to survey herself continually ... She has to survey everything she is and everything she does because how she appears to others, and ultimately how she appears to men, is of crucial importance for what is normally thought of as the success of her life. Her own sense of being in herself is supplanted by a sense of being appreciated as herself by another.

Of course, by presence, Berger means something more than physical appearance, but undoubtedly physical appearance and body image are important components.

Perhaps for society in general physical appearance has come to be overloaded with meaning. Certainly this is so for some individuals. Thus, if a plump teenager comes to feel dissatisfied with herself, perhaps for reasons which she finds difficult to define or acknowledge, she may well set out to deal with this dissatisfaction by changing her body size and shape. She will diet and the dieting will be more determined because of the extra importance it has been given. If real change in personal experience follows dieting and loss of weight, the wider importance of weight and shape will tend to be confirmed. Thus, the degree of entanglement between ideas about weight and eating control and wider personal issues will have been augmented. Certainly, it has been shown that established anorexics think about themselves and other people in ways which are dominated by concepts such as weight and shape (Crisp and Fransella, 1972). Thin and fat have come to be as pervasive concepts as good and bad or positive and negative.

Weight and body shape are ultimately controlled by eating. Eating is itself an activity which is usually invested with wide social and personal meaning over and above the fact that it is necessary to support life. It is rarely a neutral or 'matter-of-fact' issue. The psychoanalytic tradition places great emphasis upon the association of feeding and human contact in the earliest experience of the human infant. The bond between the mother and child is of central significance not only because it is, or was originally, essential for survival, but also because it is the first important relationship and forms a model for later experiences. At the basis of this primal bond is feeding. Feeding and comfort, feeding and contentment, feeding and contact, feeding and pleasure are intimately mixed from the earliest moments of infantile experience. On the other hand, feeding difficulty and hunger are associated with discomfort and displeasure. In the work of Freud and most other psycho-analytic writers the first stage of personal development is described as the oral stage and is accorded a central importance. In the language of the analyst Melanie Klein the core patterns of personal relationship are described as occurring between the person and the mother's breast, in reality for the infant and as metaphor for the adult. However, it is a metaphor which is seen as being rooted in the reality of early experience. The basic sense of self and the expectations of others are seen as being formed within the feeding relationship and emotions are first experienced in this setting. Later, in the fantasies of the unconscious, both aggression and sexuality may involve swallowing, biting and other oral activities. Of course, the mouth is not uninvolved in sex and aggression in reality. Thus from theoretical positions of this sort, it is to be expected that the actual feeding behaviour of adults, particularly disturbed adults, might provide clues to important psychological difficulties.

It is not necessary to accept the language and concepts of psycho-analysis to see that feeding may become, even for the adolescent, a loaded topic. In personal terms overeating clearly may be related to the need for comfort and a sense of reassurance. Common sense can perceive a continuity between infant feeding, thumb sucking, and overeating in times of stress. To feel that one's eating is out of control when one feels a general lack of emotional balance may easily lead to an attempt to control this feeling by imposing limits on the intake of food. Self-starvation as a means of demonstrating mastery over the demands of the body has a long history among ascetics in many cultures and religions. The symbolic element in fasting may provide an entry to a biological position which has direct physiological effects upon the drives; effects which may be welcome both to the yogi and to the anorexic. However, even without such an effect the sense of virtue which accompanies successful self-control can be very rewarding. An anorexic will often remark how dieting was an immediately positive and even pleasurable experience; she felt superior to those around her who seemed slaves to their inner impulses. While it is possible that even short-term starvation may have a subtle but pervasive influence upon brain function, explanations in purely psychological terms are probably more satisfactory.

Eating plays an important role within the enclosed world of the family and in wider social contexts. Fasting is an activity with a long history, as is the hunger strike. To eat together is an important social and family rite. To refuse to eat can be a powerful message or even a weapon. The more the family or group invests eating with meaning the more dramatic and meaningful the act of not eating becomes. There is a great number of observations which tend to suggest that the families of anorexics do indeed place greater than average importance upon food and eating (Kalucy, Crisp and Harding, 1977). The decision, for whatever reason, by a member of the family to stop eating may fall like a bombshell on such a family. The behaviour may quickly disappear as a result, but if it continues it will lead the person into a turmoil, or, perhaps, into a struggle with those who would wish to feed her. If the struggle becomes the focus of wider conflict, it may become self-perpetuating even where the original issue of slimming was not seen as of crucial importance. In Bill Naughton's play *Spring and Port Wine* the decision by the daughter of the house not to eat all of her tea-time herring quickly becomes the focus of a major family crisis. She does not become anorexic, but in real life such a situation could propel a person to abstain resolutely from food and so initiate a train of events which might end in entrapment within the condition.

Sharon was the 16-year-old daughter of a working-class household in which the evening meal was a cherished family ritual. Both parents were plump and found it difficult to sympathize with Sharon's concern about her own figure; a concern which was unremarkable among her peers. Conflict between parents and daughter about such topics as staying out too late had been simmering for some months. When Sharon went on a diet and began avoiding family mealtimes, eating became the central point at issue. A dogged resistance to the food which was pushed upon her became a matter of considerable personal importance to Sharon. She dieted with increased determination. Three or four months later she was clearly in a state of primary anorexia nervosa.

Hilde Bruch (1977, 1978) has developed a view of anorexia nervosa in which over-rigid parental expectations and the resistance of the anorexic daughter are seen as of central importance. In her book *The Golden Cage* she describes vividly families which seem to be privileged, educated and happy but who nevertheless implicitly or explicitly place upon their children the burden of living up to an ideal which is markedly constraining. These 'happy' families produce children who are described as exceptionally 'good' but who may be lacking an ability to set their own goals. Without a clear sense of their own self and their own aspirations they become over-compliant. Bruch has suggested that 'these youngsters skip the classic period of resistance early in life; they continue to function with the morality of a young child, remaining convinced of the absolute rightness of the grown ups and of their own obligation to be obedient'. Anorexia nervosa is seen as arising as an act of rebellion. Again in Bruch's words, the disorder represents 'a desperate fight against feeling enslaved and exploited, not permitted or competent to lead lives of their own. In this blind search for a sense of identity and selfhood, they will not accept anything that their parents, or the world around them, have to offer; they would rather starve than continue a life of accommodation'. This portrayal of the disorder as an act of defiance and self-preservation within these families is convincing but is open to criticism as a general model, since anorexia nervosa may be observed to arise in families and circumstances which differ very markedly from those described by Bruch. Thus, at times the parents may seem to be overtly hostile, disturbed, ill or absent and the family characterized by its chaos rather than its rigid expectations. Also the daughter may be openly rebellious and indeed feel personally impulse ridden and out of control long before the onset of the dieting which leads to the disorder.

In summary it would seem probable that a wide variety of influences may lead an individual to change her pattern of eating in order to lose weight. Perhaps in many cases the potential anorexic may begin to develop the disorder for 'normal' reasons which become distorted. These reasons may spring from her own value system or from that of her family or from the meaning which the subject has previously attached to the act of eating or to the shape of the body. Other forces may arise from the interactions between the subject and the people in her life. It seems unlikely that there is only one pattern. However, all of these roots have in common the confusion of issues about weight and eating control and other personal matters; once the anorexic career begins, this entanglement will increase because of a growing fear of losing control. Furthermore, other factors may now come to play a part.

Factors which may contribute to the continuation of anorexia nervosa

The last chapter suggested that some of the consequences of nutritional deprivation and weight loss might produce biological changes in the individual which resemble a retreat into a prepubertal state. It was suggested that the net effect of this change could be of a psychologically significant and personally relieving kind for an individual struggling with the issues of growing up. This can be thought of as a switching off or a turning down of the heat under the kettle of adolescence. Psychological and social factors, too, may be thought of as exerting an influence within the framework of adolescence.

Adolescence is by no means always a time of psychological turmoil, although it is inevitably a time of change. It is a time for testing out new behaviour and gaining new experiences. Often youthful experiment will lead to new directions for personal growth. However, many new ways will prove to lead nowhere or to places which are unacceptable to the person or those around him or her. For many individuals the process of growing towards adulthood is difficult or complicated, and it may test their ability to cope. Some form of withdrawal from the struggle is common to a number of reactions which occur around adolescence, such as drug abuse, running away and phobic behaviour. Viewed in this way anorexia nervosa is seen as another kind of withdrawal from the full force of adolescent experience. As such, it may occur most frequently where adolescence is an especially difficult or complicated process. The effect of the biological 'switching off' of puberty is likely to be relieving to the individual who feels she is failing to cope, almost regardless of the nature of the adolescent problem with which she has been struggling. There seems to be little good evidence at present that particular kinds of adolescent conflict and difficulty tend to promote the disorder over and above others. However, it is possible that an individual who especially values self-control or who comes from a family where such control is required to an unusual degree may adopt this mode of retreat in the face of trouble rather than more socially deviant ways such as drug-taking. The fact that it is first necessary to lose weight and control eating will lead anorexics to be a distorted selection of adolescents in difficulty. A range of factors may affect whether or not young people lose weight and restrict their intake sufficiently to stand a chance of entering the condition as was discussed in the previous section. It seems probable that such factors may lead to the very marked preponderance of females over males who become anorexic. If a girl or boy who is struggling with adolescent problems loses weight for any reason a withdrawal into anorexia nervosa is a risk. Once the process starts the individual may quickly become trapped by an exaggerated fear of the consequences of gaining weight. In discussing these matters it is easy to imply that the subject deliberately chooses to employ this way of coping. However, this is rarely, if ever, so. Rather, the individual finds herself in a position in which she and her experiences have changed and only then finds that to be otherwise is frightening and unacceptable.

Adolescence in its widest sense is a process which involves change in a person's experience of herself and in her relationships with others. Thus, difficulty may arise through her own failure to adapt adequately to change or through the failure of others, especially the family, to adapt appropriately. In practice these two elements tend to be closely tangled. There is a good reason for this. The features of personality which tend to influence whether or not a teenager is going to cope well with the changes of growing up are likely to have been importantly influenced in her development by her parents. Adolescence is after all simply a further stage in a process in which both parents and offspring are likely to have already influenced each other greatly. Of course, a shared genetic background will also tend to promote similarity. Thus, the child with separation anxiety at ten may well have parents who coped badly with the child's necessary separations in the past and who may have done so because of their own difficulties in this area. Such a child could well grow into a teenager with difficulties in negotiating the more major separations of adolescence and once again the parents may feel ill equipped to deal with what might be an increasingly difficult problem. It is this kind of to and fro of influence which may often make separation of the young person's difficulty from that of her parents a rather artificial task. It may be important to remember that whereas for the parents the adolescence of their daughter is a significant psychological and interpersonal process, for the daughter herself it is also a *biological* process.

Of course, not all anorexic subjects are adolescent in the narrower sense of the word; that is, they have not all gone through puberty in recent years. However, it is possible that for those individuals who fall ill at a later age the issues of adolescence are still unresolved in some way. Many older anorexics have difficulties which resemble those of younger sufferers in managing matters such as their sexuality, their impulses or problems of dependence and independence. It could be that these older individuals also retain a capacity to 'switch off' biologically which is greater than that of their peers, but such a suggestion is at present pure speculation.

For once it may be appropriate to use the example of a male anorexic to illustrate the kind of changes which seem to be brought about by the alteration of weight in anorexic subjects.

Keith was aged twenty-eight at the time of his admission for treatment and had been suffering from primary anorexia nervosa for about nine years. He had previously consulted physicians and a psychiatrist and had been diagnosed variously. However, he had a clearly established weight phobia which led him to keep his weight at least 28 per cent below a normal level by means of abstinence, an odd diet and occasional vomiting. He was the only child of a soldier who had been largely absent from home until Keith was aged five. His mother, an anxious and insecure woman, had established an extremely close and exclusive relationship with her little boy; for instance, she slept in the same bed with him. When father returned home this sleeping arrangement continued for a further four years and effectively ended the parents' sexual life together. Keith grew up an anxious boy who was, however, inclined to be quick-tempered and impulsive. In his late teens he joined the army in a bid for independence but began drinking heavily. He was already a plump young man and he put on more weight. On leave he met and quickly became engaged to a girl of whom his mother, perhaps surprisingly, approved. He was bought out of the army and went on a diet prior to his wedding. The marriage was not consummated and the couple parted after a year. In retrospect it seems clear that Keith had been anorexic since the time of his marriage or just before. He continued to live on alone working steadily but unhappily at a clerical job. He rarely went out except to visit his parents and he did not drink. Occasionally he would consult doctors, mainly about odd physical complaints, and was eventually diagnosed as having anorexia nervosa. He was offered in-patient treatment at the psychiatric unit of a London teaching hospital and, with mixed feelings, he accepted. Treatment comprised a strict regime of bed rest and weight restoration together with individual psychotherapy. His mother was interviewed but was not involved in the treatment to any substantial extent. As Keith put on weight a marked change occurred. At first he had been quiet and compliant. His hair was cut very short and he shaved twice daily because of his dislike for the 'dirty' appearance which resulted from his rather swarthy complexion. However, as the weeks went by and his weight approached more normal levels he became more assertive and at times rather rebellious. His temper became evident and he began talking of rather unrealistic plans for a new life. His appearance altered in parallel with his new ideas about himself. He allowed his hair to grow and he was soon sporting a Zapata-style moustache. After he had attained a strictly average body weight for his age and height, he was allowed increasing freedom prior to his discharge from hospital. On at least one occasion he returned to the hospital drunk and eventually he left rather sooner than was ideal and against advice. Subsequently, he maintained rather erratic contact with his psychiatrist and often missed appointments. He returned to his old job but now attempted to lead a busy social life. He did not see his parents. Increasingly his life came to be centred around heavy drinking, at first with others and then alone. He said that alcohol gave him confidence. Within three months of his leaving hospital his weight had begun to fall. After a further three months he was once again very thin, had given up drinking, had resumed visiting his parents and had shaved off his moustache. He wrote a letter saying that he did not want any further contact with the hospital.

An understanding of Keith's story would suggest that the anorexia nervosa had resolved much of his late adolescent conflict by quenching the biological basis of his adulthood. His rebellious, impulse-ridden behaviour and the consequent anxiety were thus contained although at the expense of his sexual capacity and perhaps his vitality in general. These were rekindled with weight restoration but so were the old conflicts. He failed to find a new and more satisfactory resolution and, therefore, relapsed. The treatment alliance proved inadequate for the task of providing a secure yet permissive space in which he could find new ways of coping. His rebelliousness, which undoubtedly had its roots in the relationship with his parents, was transferred into his relationship with those who were trying to help him and disrupted it. Of course, it could be argued that the psychological aspects of the treatment programme were solely responsible for the remarkable change which occurred but on balance it seems more likely that the biological consequences of weight change were of central importance. Certainly Keith saw weight as having considerable personal significance. His story illustrates dramatically the changes in style and apparent personality which may parallel weight change in anorexia nervosa. The changes were clear and obvious because they involved his behaviour and appearance. Similar changes in other cases may be much less obvious to the observer and yet may nevertheless be experienced profoundly but coped with quietly by the anorexic.

It is not difficult to think of circumstances which might make growing up more difficult. Examples could include parental psychiatric illness, parental strife, parental loss, disturbance in elder siblings, or major family crises. Clinical experience and relevant literature tend to confirm that these are indeed commonly found in the background of young people with the disorder (Kalucy, Crisp and Harding, 1977). Furthermore, there is evidence that adverse sexual experiences, often occurring in childhood and of a very disturbing kind, frequently appear in the histories of anorexic patients (Oppenheimer *et al.*, 1985). Often, however, it takes a good deal of detailed knowledge of an anorexic's own view of her world to see the difficulties which confront her. Frequently such knowledge is kept hidden by the anorexic or revealed only partially or slowly to a skilful interviewer whom she has come to trust. Such investigation is open to the criticism that the investigator may read into everyday situations all manner of troubles, but nevertheless such sensitive listening and reconstruction of the world view of another is a central feature of clinical method.

Once an individual is established in a state of anorexia nervosa her behaviour will change and usually she will come to be treated differently by others. There will be an adjustment in the mutual expectations which she shares with those around her. She will come to occupy a different role. Often she will move into some form of sick role, but the anorexic does not usually behave as a 'good' sick person should. She may be willing to lay aside some of her usual responsibilities and obligations, she may welcome the care and concern of others, but she will not often be seen to seek help which would lead to her recovery. The prospect of change is too frightening for her, and the disorder may, in a sense, be serving a purpose in enabling her to cope, albeit within a constricted and limited range. The notion of a new role implies that other actors in her personal circle will have also changed their parts. Often this will involve an increase in conflict as the people around the anorexic try to get her to change. Sometimes, however, the onset of the disorder and the role changes which it brings lead to a reduction in conflict. It may be not only some sort of solution to the turmoil of the anorexic individual but it may also bring relief to those who are close to her through changes in relationships. When this occurs the trap of anorexia nervosa will be secured with greater force.

Anne was 17 years old and at secretarial college when she developed anorexia nervosa. She had put on weight rapidly over the previous year because of relative overeating which

seemed to be her way of comforting herself in her unhappiness. She had gone on a slimming diet and quickly lost a lot of weight. She became weak and complained that any attempt to eat substantial quantities of food led her to feel bloated and sick. Increasingly she would avoid going out, gave up college and stayed at home pottering about in her dressing-gown or even staying in bed.

There was more than one cause of her unhappiness, but a major problem was the rift between her parents. For several years her father, a salesman, had been having an affair with a woman who was considerably younger than himself and his wife. Anne had known of this for some time and indeed about two years before she developed anorexia nervosa, her father had left home but returned after a few weeks. Several months before Anne fell ill, he had, however, left again saying that this time it was for good. Anne had always been especially close to her father and she missed him a great deal. When he visited the family home there was talk of Anne, once she was finished at college, going to live with her father and his girlfriend. Anne's mother was depressed and bitterly hurt by her husband's behaviour. She said that she felt that her life was over when he left her and still hoped that one day he would come back to live with her. However, she remained angry and found it difficult to tolerate comments from her children or others which seemed to excuse her husband or minimize her suffering. Anne was the middle of three children. Her 19-year-old brother tended to cut himself off from the family and her 14-year-old sister was the most studious and academically successful member of the family.

After her parents' separation Anne found herself to be full of strong but conflicting feelings. She felt that she could under-stand both her mother and her father, but such a neutral posi-tion was difficult to sustain. Both parents separately confided in her and sought her as an ally. She tended to feel disloyal to both of them. Her brother and sister were of little help to her. Likewise, a relationship with a boyfriend gave her little support and indeed presented her with problems about how she should manage her own sexuality which seemed the more difficult because of the contradictory examples given by her parents.

In due course Anne's anorexic behaviour was recognized as

an illness by the family, and the resulting shifts in relationship were in some ways simplifying and relieving for both Anne and her parents. Thus Anne's mother found a new purpose in looking after her sick daughter. Furthermore, she became unequivocally the object of consolation and support from her friends. She blamed her husband explicitly for her daughter's illness, but nevertheless felt that concern for their daughter was something that he shared with her but not with his girl-friend. The father in his turn had a reason to visit the household and could expiate his guilt by proper concern for his sick child. Anne herself felt able to accept passively the appropriate atten-tions of both parents and she could avoid the need for any action which could be construed as taking sides. The need for their love, her anger at their behaviour and her wish for her parents to be together again all somehow found expression in her illness and the changes which followed it. Likewise, the thornier problems of life were postponed to an unspecified time in the future when she would be well.

In this case, it should not be thought that Anne did not suffer discomfort and distress as a result of her anorexic state nor that her parents did not worry about her and wish her well. Rather the continuing distress of all parties was made simpler and more manage-able by the illness. The conflicting emotions of the whole family could at least in part find a common direction and perhaps a common enemy in the form of the ill health that had overtaken Anne. In subtle ways, such a state of affairs not uncommonly leads to an undermining of attempts by others to help the anorexic to recover. The path out of the condition becomes more of an uphill struggle.

6 · Treatments

It is possible to view anorexia nervosa as a way of coping, but it is undoubtedly a maladaptive way. The disadvantages of remaining within the condition are obvious to others and are directly experienced by the anorexic. It is not that she is immune to the miseries which self-starvation brings, but rather that from her point of view they are outweighed by the fear of change. Just as the agoraphobic housewife is willing to bear the restrictions of life in one place rather than face her terror of going out, so the girl with anorexia nervosa restricts her diet, her body and her experience, rather than face the consequences of not doing so which have come to seem so frightening to her. Inevitably the anorexic will be ambivalent about attempts to help her. Sometimes her current suffering will seem a greater burden than the risks of change, and she will struggle to put on weight. Sometimes she will succeed, but more often an initial small gain will lead to a strengthening of her fear and the old pattern will be resumed. Those around her will urge her to eat, but sooner or later they will begin to advise her to seek professional help. It is usually medical help which is sought. Her family and friends will have started to construe the problem as an illness; a state beyond the powers of everyday persuasion.

This chapter will attempt to outline the consequences for the anorexic subject of becoming a patient. It will concentrate on medical services although, of course, some anorexics escape from their condition without professional intervention, and others derive help from teachers, social workers, clergymen, lay therapists and others.

Presentation to medical care

Not all anorexic subjects see doctors. A significant minority, even of the most severely ill, manage to avoid any kind of medical assessment or care. However, most sufferers from anorexia nervosa do eventually come into contact with medical services. Many, however, present themselves to doctors only following pressure from their relatives and others, and with at least some show of resistance. The anorexic will typically have mixed feelings about seeking help and this will show itself in different ways. Clearly a girl in her early teens is more likely to be bundled along to the doctor than is the woman in her twenties living alone. The older woman's ambivalence may, perhaps, be shown by the presentation for medical help of a single symptom such as insomnia, amenorrhoea or constipation. Typically, it is to her family doctor that the anorexic will find her way first.

The late Dr Michael Balint in his writings on interactions in medical practice has described the way in which the patient makes an 'offer' of a symptom or illness which then becomes the subject of negotiation with the doctor until an 'agreement' has been reached as to how it shall be considered (Balint, 1964). Such language is relevant to the varied ways in which anorexia nervosa is perceived and talked about. Thus the woman who presents complaining of a sleep problem may welcome a premature closure of discussion and leave the surgery with her sleeping pills, relieved for the moment that her thinness was not remarked upon. From the doctor's point of view, a diagnosis of anorexia nervosa may not have been considered, or if it was, it may have been too readily dismissed as either improbable or, as a Pandora's box of problems, best left alone. Certainly, except in extreme cases, not all doctors will readily consider anorexia nervosa as a diagnosis. Many have had little experience of or teaching about the disorder and may consider it an unimportant rarity. Others fail to distinguish it from the background of concern about weight and shape which they rightly feel to be the norm among young women. The behaviour of an anorexic can seem silly and even perverse, and the doctor may be antagonized by her reluctance to be straightforward about her condition. An ambivalent patient may accentuate the mixed feelings of the doctor and her childishness may bring out the finger-wagging parent in him. Even at this early stage, relationships have a tendency to become complicated. The 'offer' of the patient is normally not a simple one and the response of the doctor will need to be carefully tuned if an appropriate 'agreement' is to be reached. What might this 'agreement' be?

A markedly thin woman in her early twenties presenting with constipation arouses her doctor's suspicion enough to inquire about menstruation, diet and weight. She initially answers that her periods are 'irregular' and her appetite is 'all right'. A little persistence, however, produces the information that she has not had a period for eight months and eats only one meal of green salad each day. She refuses to be weighed, but her refusal is used by the doctor as a 'way in' to asking her about her attitudes to weight. She becomes tearful and un-forthcoming, but there is a silent acknowledgement that this is a problem area. The doctor puts it into words. He says that he suspects that weight has become very important to her and that she is frightened by the way she feels, but even more frightened of eating more or putting on weight. She nods, but says that she feels bloated after eating and feels she could eat more if she wasn't constipated. The doctor accepts for the moment this level of disclosure and does not push her further. He says that he feels that the problem is more com-plicated than simple constipation and that he does not think it would be appropriate to prescribe a laxative at this stage. He says that he would like to do a blood test and see her again to discuss things further in a week's time. He takes blood for a haemoglobin and erythrocyte sedimentation rate (a simple screening test for a variety of physical diseases) and for electrolyte estimation (a low serum potassium would suggest habitual vomiting or laxative abuse). Doctor and patient have not reached a final 'agreement', but some pro-gress has been made and a premature closure of the matter has been avoided. The doctor, while acknowledging his concern for the physical aspects of the problem, has not taken the patient's 'offer' at face value; the patient, while not abandoning her emphasis on her bowels, has allowed the discussion to widen to include her weight and diet in the problem. At her next visit, she may well feel able to talk more fully.

Aims of treatment

When an agreement, even a provisional one, has been reached

between doctor and patient, it becomes necessary to make a treatment plan. The general practitioner will decide whether to proceed or to seek specialist help. Either way, the aims of the treatment may be stated as being (i) the restoration of both a normal weight and an adequate, balanced diet, and (ii) psychological readjustment, including the diminution and eventual loss of the 'weight phobia'.

There is no clear consensus as to how these aims should be achieved. The eventual balance between attention to the physical and the psychological will be determined by the attitude and views of both doctor and patient, and by their agreement. In cases where the anorexic is young, the parents and others may also influence what happens. If both parties emphasize the physical, they may come to talk together about the anorexia nervosa as being an 'inability to tolerate food' and the treatment as being to 'retrain the stomach to take an adequate diet'. If specialist referral is decided upon, it will be to a physician rather than a psychiatrist. Of course, the specialist and the patient have to reach a fresh 'agreement' which will, however, be influenced on the patient's side by her earlier contact with the general practitioner. Moreover, many family doctors who know the available specialists well will have tended to refer their patient to a consultant whom they anticipate will have views and attitudes not too greatly at odds with their own. What may be considered an over-emphasis of the physical may occur when the anorexic subject, or those around her, cannot tolerate the thought that emotional disorder may be involved; these views may be especially prevalent among those who fall ill in this way. Furthermore, many doctors feel more comfortable dealing with physical illness, and some may be happy to go along with a playing down of the psychological aspects. Conversely, an emphasis on the emotional may occur when the patient is able to talk about her feelings and her relationships, and perhaps does so in part as a 'smoke screen' to avoid too much attention to the painful area of weight and its significance. The doctor may hold the view that disturbed emotional development and personal relationships are basic to the disorder and may collude with a shelving of the weight issue in the belief that he is 'getting to the bottom of things'. If specialist referral occurs it will be to obtain psychiatric help, and unfortunately the collusion may sometimes be continued within the relationship between the patient and her psychiatrist.

What is the correct balance between attention to the physical and psychological? It would seem clear that changes in both aspects must occur if the individual is to have an opportunity to recover fully. Indeed, the dichotomy seems artificial if recovery is viewed as a change from one stable, albeit maladaptive, psychological position to another which is more satisfactory. Both parts of the task are of equal importance, although individuals may vary as to the amount of help of each kind they require. The majority needs substantial aid towards the accomplishment of both aims. The best approach to treatment occurs when doctor and patient are able to include in their 'agreement' some shared understanding of the whole task. Then it becomes possible for them to make a more or less explicit contract outlining what each is undertaking. Sometimes this may even take written form, and often the family of a younger patient will need to be involved.

At the end of a lengthy out-patient assessment, a 17-year-old girl with gross weight loss and a predominantly abstinent eating pattern is able to make an informal contract with her psychiatrist about the admission to hospital that is being planned. She has described her great fear that once she starts eating she will be unable to stop. She is also very worried about her widowed mother who has recently been considerably depressed. She is frightened of upsetting her more and argues that her admission to hospital may do this. The psychiatrist suspects that she fears a more general loss of control if she abandons her present position. It is this more pervasive threat to her ability to be a good daughter which she dreads as being harmful to her mother. She worries greatly about the mother and, of course, the mother worries about her. These matters are discussed, although at every opportunity the girl returns doggedly to talking about her fear of eating. She seems reassured when it is agreed that her mother will be involved in regular discussions throughout her admission. The treatment is explained as being aimed at restoring her to a weight normal for her age and height, and that she will be expected to eat the mixed diet provided. Everyone will be as concerned to stop her overeating as they are to see that she feeds herself adequately. The regime is described in some detail and the psychiatrist emphasizes that as she gains weight she may feel mixed up and bewildered, but that in hospital she will have the opportunity to talk regularly about how she feels with someone who is used to helping people in this way. The girl agrees to go into hospital on these terms. She has been surprised at the degree to which her fears have been understood and even anticipated by the doctor. However, she has unspoken reservations about the enterprise and is reassured by the thought that if the promised help doesn't work out, she can always discharge herself. As she leaves the consulting room she asks for one further assurance that she will be stopped if she starts overeating.

The idea of a contract demands an opportunity for discussion before treatment is started, and requires circumstances in which each party feels free to decide not to enter into treatment if both cannot agree to its terms. Clearly when the patient is extremely ill neither of these conditions may apply. A third aim may then be added; that is, to save the patient's life. Usually in these circumstances the anorexic subject will at least acquiesce to measures aimed at stabilizing her physical state. Occasionally the responsible clinician may feel justified in detaining a patient for such treatment under the provisions of the Mental Health Act. However, such a course must be the last resort in an extreme situation and its use may complicate the subsequent relationship with the patient. Indeed, in practice compulsion is very rarely justified. Its use goes against the need for the patient, with help, to take responsibility for herself, which is a crucial element of eventual success. Certainly, once the physical danger is past, there will be a need to consider a contract for further treatment. A degree of mutual trust and co-operation may be difficult to obtain, but is an important foundation for success in the treatment of anorexia nervosa.

Weight restoration

All authorities agree that restoration of a more normal body weight must occur if someone is to recover from anorexia nervosa. Indeed, some would seem in practice to regard this as the only aim. However, opinions as to how the patient is to be helped to achieve this aim vary considerably. Also, as has been emphasized above, not all patients will require or accept the same amount of help. Furthermore, some subjects may find it more difficult to stabilize at a satisfactory weight or to maintain a balanced diet than to regain a normal body weight in the first place. Merely to regain weight is, at best, half the battle.

At the least, an anorexic subject will require encouragement and advice. Occasionally this is all that is needed when she presents at a stage when she is already struggling to put on weight. She will then usually be helped by the provision of a clear framework in which she can continue her struggle, while perhaps more attention is paid to the emotional context of her illness. Such a framework can often be provided by a general practitioner or by a psychiatrist or other specialist on an out-patient basis. There is little that is essentially medical about the task in these circumstances and other professions may appropriately undertake it. The nature and constituents of supportive help are more difficult to describe and define than those of more active treatment. The need for at least an implicit contract is no less important here. Thus, it is useful at an early stage to define a target weight towards which the anorexic is aiming. Indeed, such a weight may be useful in all circumstances. If it is taken explicitly from the available tables of average weight by height, age and sex, this may go a little way to convince the patient that the doctor does not have unduly distorted views on what weight is ideal. Unavoidably, the subject will be able to bring up many examples of her healthy contemporaries who are markedly lighter than the average weights of the tables. In general it may, none the less, be best to settle on a strictly average weight. However, in some circumstances, for instance, when the girl has been ill for some years and has never in her life been as heavy as the average weight for her current age and height, it may be appropriate to agree upon a lighter weight, perhaps that shown as average for the age at which she fell ill.

It will be important that the doctor sees the anorexic subject regularly throughout her attempt at weight gain, which may take many weeks or months. He will need to weigh her and review her progress in modifying her diet. A mixed balanced diet, including carbohydrate, eaten at conventional mealtimes, is desirable. However, the doctor may sometimes think it best to advise a patient who is over-enthusiastically aiming at too rapid a weight gain by eating an extreme or distorted diet to reduce her intake. The dangers here are that the eating may get out of control, that it may lead to a panic, and that this will in turn lead to giving up the attempt. Furthermore, such overeating is hardly good practice for the stability of both weight and diet, which is the aim once a normal weight has been restored. The anorexic may need simple advice on what is an appropriate diet. The range of eating patterns in the general population is wide, but the doctor should realize that it may have been years since the subject ate simply to maintain a stable adult weight or that she may never have done so. In some circumstances, particularly where 'bingeing' has been a problem, it may be useful for the patient to record everything she eats in a special diary. If spaces are ruled out for each meal on the daily pages, this will make clear the difference between meals and 'pickings'. The diary can be reviewed by the therapist and patient together at their meetings. 'Rewards' and 'punishments' may be made contingent on changes in eating behaviour and weight if both parties have agreed to this, but clearly such a behavioural approach is more easily arranged in the controlled setting of in-patient treatment. However, significant reward and punishment may arise from the approval or disapproval of the doctor and the reaction of the patient herself when she reviews her own behaviour with him. All in all, the elements of continuity, of understanding and support which the doctor can provide for the patient may be most powerful in helping her in her fight to change. There is, of course, no clear borderline between this role of sympathetic supervisor of weight and diet, and the more clearly psychotherapeutic role which will be discussed in the next section.

Successful intervention in the course of many cases of established anorexia nervosa requires in-patient treatment. This will usually mean the referral of the patient from the general practitioner to the care of a hospital consultant. The type of specialist who undertakes such treatment is usually a psychiatrist or a physician, often one who is especially concerned with disorders of hormonal function (endocrinologist) or of the digestive system (gastroenterologist). Other hospital doctors may have anorexic patients referred to them from time to time, e.g., gynaecologists because of the amenorrhoea, or neurologists because of fits; they will, however, only rarely undertake the complete treatment of the disorder.

The style and emphasis of the treatment offered once the patient is admitted will vary considerably, both between specialities and between individual clinicians within the specialities. Just as there is no clear consensus as to the nature of anorexia nervosa, so there is no uniformity of treatment; even of treatment aimed at the limited target of weight restoration. Basic to most treatment regimes, however, are the persuasive and supportive powers of those whose task it is to supervise immediately the patient's eating. This will almost always be the nursing staff. Their role is both crucial to the patient's progress and demanding of their skills. The task of persuading a reluctant patient to eat is never an easy one and can be distressing to the nurse when the anorexic weeps, shouts, or otherwise behaves like a persecuted child. A female nurse may herself have dieted in the past or be currently slimming, and may be torn between empathy for the anorexic's fear of becoming fat and annoyance at her childish behaviour. The nurse's ability to act in a sympathetic yet firm manner will be enhanced if she too has a shared understanding of the nature of the anorexic's plight and a knowledge of the contract of treatment. Where there is no clear contract, the patient may well be able to play off nurse against doctor, or nurse against nurse in a way which is not helpful and may ultimately lead to a frightening loss of security and trust.

The nurse's task is to convey a simple and yet resolute expectation that the patient should eat, and to do this in spite of all the attempts of the patient to widen or otherwise change the issue. This is not to say that the nurse will not talk about anything but food; the job is rather to keep feeding and other topics apart. This is a difficult task, but it is somewhat easier for the professional nurse than for the parents of an anorexic daughter. For them such a separation may be almost impossible. Sir William Gull was approaching the same point when he wrote, 'Patients should be fed at regular intervals and surrounded by persons who would have moral control over them; relatives and friends being generally the worst attendants'.

In extreme cases, spoon-feeding or even tube-feeding may be practised, but these techniques should rarely be necessary.

Surprisingly, a few authors have advocated their regular use (Groen and Feldman-Toledano, 1966), but, in general, a situation in which they are even considered indicates a failure to engage the subject in a treatment contract or a failure of nursing technique, or both. It must be admitted, however, that failure is relative to the task and, occasionally, both the medical and nursing tasks may seem almost impossibly difficult.

Usually the nursing and medical efforts directed toward helping the patient to regain weight are organized into a clearly defined package or regime. In centres where many such patients are treated, this regime tends to become well known to all those involved and constitutes a 'culture' which can provide a secure base for both staff and patients. Where an individual anorexic is managed on a ward where such patients are uncommon, such an atmosphere is much more difficult to achieve. Most clinicians would agree that patients, relatives and staff should know what to expect. Ideally, the features of the treatment regime should be made clear from the outset and combined in a contract with the proposed psychological help. Measures which seem punitive when imposed without explanation upon a bewildered and resisting patient may actually become reassuring when they are presented as part of a regime whose purpose is to provide a sufficiently secure setting for a struggle to change. For instance, it is a common feature of many regimes to oblige the patient to use a bedpan or commode rather than the ward lavatory and also for the wash-basin to be blocked up. Both these measures are designed to prevent, or at least to make obvious, attempts to dispose of uneaten food or vomit. If the ward staff explain these actions appropriately to their patient, she will usually accept or even welcome them. Certainly, nothing is gained by disguising or hiding the purpose of these rules and limitations. The anorexic may be upset or affronted at first, but she will be reassured if the doctors and nurses can help her to cope successfully with the panic which comes when routes for 'psychological escape' are blocked.

A planned regime for weight gain needs to state how much weight is to be gained, by means of what diet and in what circumstances. The idea of defining a target weight has already been discussed in connection with out-patient management. It is an important strategy in hospital also. Where it is used, the timing of discharge will normally be determined by the subject reaching this weight. It may not be best, however, for the anorexic to be discharged immediately following the attainment of her target. Attaining a weight is one thing, maintaining it is another. A period for readjustment of diet and attitude may be valuable. Once a target weight is defined, the speed with which the patient reaches it will depend upon how much she eats. The size of the diet which is advocated will be the result of a compromise between a wish not to prolong unduly the period of weight restoration and the opposing desire to avoid a diet so heavy that it is unacceptable to the patient. Also, eating very large amounts provides a poor model for future normal eating. Most authors agree that the diet should be mixed to include protein, fat and carbohydrate. Different treatment regimes will include different diets. Thus Dally suggested in 1969 that the in-patient should increase her intake over the first week or two of admission until an intake of 4,000 to 5,000 calories per day is reached. Likewise, in 1970 Russell advocated a diet giving up to 5,000 calories per day. Such high figures are obtained with the aid of high-calorie drinks which are used either as the mainstay or as adjuncts to normal food. Crisp, on the other hand, has argued against the use of very special diets, and in-patients under his care receive a substantial, but commonplace, hospital diet giving between 2,500 and 3,000 calories per day. The upper limit is especially enforced so as to provide the patient with a sense of external control of any impulse to overeat (Crisp, 1967). Lucas and his colleagues in the United States advocate a small diet 'calculated to maintain the admission weight' which is only gradually increased to promote weight gain (Lucas, Duncan and Piens, 1976). Such differences of recommended diet are a matter of style and emphasis; in the absence of comparative studies, a middle-of-the-road position would seem to be sensible. However, everyone involved should realize that a substantial weight deficit of, for example, 33 lb (15 kg) will take many weeks or even months to restore.

Some limitation of activity is a part of most treatment regimes. Sometimes the anorexic is nursed in a single room and expected to stay in or on her bed for twenty-four hours per day. She may not leave the room for any purpose. A commode or bedpan is used. Such a regime may seem punitive, but many anorexic patients come to feel safe and secure within their 'cell'. Bed rest has been recommended in the treatment of anorexia nervosa for many decades and has been construed variously as necessary to support a weakened and sedated patient, to cut energy use and hence promote weight gain, or as a device to aid nursing control and observation. Bed rest represents in a clear way the dependency of the patient which is a more or less explicit feature of most treatment programmes. In the beginning, the staff may be actively seeking to encourage such dependency and will want control over the patient's behaviour. Later they will wish to hand back this control to the patient and encourage her autonomy. Such a transition is difficult to achieve and may be facilitated in some regimes by a gradual and almost ritualized remobilization from complete bed rest. Even if the change is thought about by all concerned mainly in physical terms, it is none the less an important process in the psychological readjustment of the anorexic under treatment.

Some programmes are organized so that treatment can be altered in a graduated way to reward the patient for desired behaviour. Allowing the patient to get up more as weight is gained is a commonplace feature of treatment regimes. However, some workers have devised management programmes in which reward ('reinforcement') is made contingent on either weight gain or satisfactory eating. For instance, Bhanji and Thompson, working at Guy's Hospital, London, described in 1974 a regime in which finishing the meal in a certain time was reinforced by an individually devised system of rewards which included being allowed letters, visitors, newspapers and so on. The detailed co-operation of the patient and her relatives was required, since at first the anorexic was isolated in a single room with only essential furnishing and limited contact with the nursing staff, and had to 'earn' her access to a more satisfying situation. Interestingly, Bhanji and Thompson did not let their patients know their weights, whereas others have devised similar regimes using weight gain as the behaviour to be reinforced (Eckert *et al.*, 1979). On the whole, little advantage has been found in strict behavioural regimes and their use would seem to be declining. Minuchin and his colleagues in Philadelphia have combined such behaviour therapy with family therapy in a programme which starts with a fairly brief hospital admission (two to three weeks) during which a behavioural regime is introduced in which activity is made contingent upon weight gain (Minuchin, Rosman and Baker, 1978). The family is involved early on in the treatment regime by the use of family therapy lunch sessions in which the problems of the patient and the family are discussed in the context of a shared meal. After discharge, therapy is continued in modified form with the aim of not only restoring weight, but also of restructuring the family system. Their treatment programme is clearly an integrated one and has some interesting and novel features. It is, however, applicable mainly to young patients who are still in the care of their family and, of course, requires the family to co-operate closely in treatment.

The place of drugs in the management of primary anorexia nervosa is another matter upon which there is no clear consensus. However, most authorities would agree that their role is not essential or at best they may form just a part of a treatment programme. Over the last decade or so, the most extensively used drug has been chlorpromazine. This is a major tranquillizer or neuroleptic of the phenothiazine group, which is widely used in psychiatry for the treatment of psychotic states, particularly acute schizophrenia. Here it usually has the effect of not only calming the patient, but also of reducing the distressing perceptual changes and disorders of the form of thought which characterize such disorders. Its use in the treatment of anorexia nervosa was first reported by Dally and Sargant in 1960, and it has become a feature of many treatment regimes since that time. Its mode of action would seem to be best thought of as the promotion of sedation and a calmer state of mind which may tend to allow the anorexic to co-operate more fully with other aspects of treatment and, in particular, to eat a full diet. It is also useful where restlessness reduces compliance with a regime which demands bed rest. It seems unlikely that the value of chlorpromazine depends on any more specific mechanism. Where restlessness is not a major problem and a reasonable therapeutic alliance has been established between the patient and her doctor, the role of chlorpromazine and similar drugs would seem to be small. Cyproheptadine, an appetite-stimulating drug, may have some place in the management of selected patients (Goldberg *et al.*, 1979).

In their influential paper of 1960, Dally and Sargant advocated the use of insulin in conjunction with chlorpromazine. Insulin is the hormone which is deficient in diabetes mellitus. It has an effect on metabolism which tends to promote a lowering of blood sugar. Insulin therapy has been used in the treatment of anorexia nervosa because it tends to promote a readiness to eat a substantial meal. The experience of such a procedure need not be unpleasant and is usually accompanied by considerable individual attention and concern from the nursing staff. However, its basic rationale is to increase appetite and this may often miss the point in the management of those patients who, far from lacking appetite, are engaged in a constant struggle against a desire to eat which, at least to them, seems frighteningly insatiable. In such patients it is possible that insulin therapy may tend to encourage a tendency toward overeating. It is a treatment which needs to be carefully managed if it is to be safe and, on balance, it probably offers little benefit which cannot be gained in other ways. It is now hardly ever used.

Antidepressant drugs and even electroconvulsive therapy have been used in the treatment of anorexia nervosa, usually because the clinician concerned has thought of the disorder as a variant of depressive illness. Most authorities would, however, reject both this view and its implications for treatment. From time to time, a wide variety of other drugs have been advocated, but usually on the basis of slender evidence, and the verdict on their usefulness must be one of 'not proven'. In general the place of drugs in the treatment of anorexia nervosa today is about the same as that described by Gull in 1873. He wrote that 'the author had not observed much advantage from the administration of drugs whether tonics or alternatives. Believing the disorder to be due to want of mental equilibrium, he would rather trust to moral influences and to feeding than to medicines, though these might still be amongst the *adjuvantia*'.

In summary then it may be said that a number of treatment regimes have been designed and used to help the anorexic to gain weight. Common to most of them are rest, and the careful supervision of feeding. Common to all of them, however, is the desirability of an adequate level of co-operation between the anorexic patient and those who are trying to help her. There is a lack of good comparative studies of different treatment regimes, but it may well be that success depends less upon the details of a regime than upon the extent to which it is enthusiastically and thoroughly carried out. The anorexic who is gaining weight in hospital is facing a change in herself which she has come to dread. Only the patient can eat the necessary food, only she feels the discomfort and panic which eating may bring and only she can feel what it is like to experience such a rapid change in body size. However, the presence around her of a team who seem to know what they are doing, why they are doing it and the effects treatment is having upon her will tend to allow the patient to make best use of whatever courage and motivation she possesses.

Psychological help

However much attention is paid to the physical aspects of treatment, the process of change which it may bring about is a highly emotional experience for the anorexic. Whether or not she relapses will depend upon her ability to cope with this experience. Thus, treatment which is solely directed toward weight restoration will, if successful, give the subject an opportunity to make a full recovery, but the opportunity will be of a 'sink or swim' kind; the anorexic will be given no special help to exploit the opportunity to make a different adjustment. In practice, of course, she may well use aspects of the treatment regime to help herself emotionally, even if such help is informal and not part of the planned programme. Thus a teenage patient may derive help from chatting to a nearly contemporary student nurse, although neither may construe it as treatment. A discussion which starts with the discovery of a shared interest in music may allow the patient to use the nurse as a source of information about how others cope with the common concerns of adolescence. Psychological help alone, on the other hand, will not provide such an opportunity for useful change unless it leads indirectly to weight gain. Much time can be spent in psychotherapy without weight gain being achieved. The exercise will usually be a sterile one for all concerned as long as the physical position of the subject remains firmly an anorexic one. Weight restoration may not be a sufficient cause for recovery, but it is a necessary one. While the same may be said of psychological readjustment, the nature of the required change is variable and certainly difficult to define. In the absence of firm evidence and the power to predict outcome, there is a danger of slipping into a circular argument. That is, true recovery takes place only when psychological readjustment occurs and when the patient does not recover it is evidence that such readjustment has not happened. It could be that there are indicators of real change of a psychological kind which would prove as useful in predicting recovery as weight gain is on the physical side, but they are as yet undocumented. In the meantime, practical clinicians must use whatever clues they can in making a judgement about their patient's psychological state. In practice, when an anorexic has regained a normal weight and she and her doctor are reasonably sure that she has also changed psychologically, only time will tell if they are right. The doctor's predictions may usually be correct, but even the most experienced practitioner will sometimes be surprised by a patient who either recovers or relapses in a quite unexpected way. Perhaps it is this elusive character of the psychological elements of anorexia nervosa and its treatment which makes some doctors shy away from becoming intentionally involved in this aspect of their patient's care. That something is difficult to measure, however, does not mean that it is unreal or unimportant. Nor is it possible for the clinician to avoid influencing the patient's emotional life. Indeed, the emotional transition which weight restoration promotes may be such that the person undergoing it is particularly open to influence for better or worse. Likewise, the dependence which most treatment regimes enforce upon their subjects may make those in control of these regimes especially influential.

Many regimes deliberately set out to exploit this influential position in a number of ways. Ideally perhaps all members of the treatment team should see their role as involving the emotional support of the patient, but often one individual is made especially available to the anorexic for regular discussion. This individual, or the person who is seen as being in charge of the treatment, or both, may come to seem especially important to the patient in a way which can perhaps be best understood in terms of the psychoanalytic concept of transference. This concept has a number of related definitions, but in general it denotes the patient's perception of current figures in her life, particularly that of her therapist,

which is profoundly influenced by feelings and attitudes transferred
from earlier important relationships, particularly that with her
parents. It is hardly surprising that a young person who is
undergoing a contrived and accelerated process of 'growing up' as
weight is gained may come to display transference-related behaviour toward those who are importantly involved in bringing
this process about. How this transference is managed can vary
considerably. In the special circumstances of psychoanalysis,
transference phenomena are selectively pointed out or 'interpreted'
to the patient in order to promote insight. Such interpretation is
only one of several options open, and in the context of most
treatment regimes for anorexia nervosa it is often not the most
appropriate. Direct discussion of the transference is a technique
which can quickly lead the unwary therapist into waters in which
he feels out of his depth. Alternative techniques involve the use of
the concept of transference in ways which stop short of interpretation. Thus such ideas might aid in the doctor's understanding
of his patient's reactions and allow him to respond appropriately.
The therapist's response may be in accordance with the transferred
role or opposed to it, or more likely, simply follow a line which
emphasizes the realities of the situation, without becoming 'sucked
in' unduly by the inappropriate demands of the patient. The therapist's interventions will be determined by his own emotional response (counter-transference), and in 1967 Crisp emphasized that it
is important for the therapist to be aware of and to control the
counter-transference in order to provide the patient with an appropriate and secure interpersonal relationship. Often this may
involve a solid defence of the rationale of the regime combined with
a considerable capacity to listen and reflect without loading the
patient with directive advice about her life in general. The individual therapist in an in-patient situation may, therefore, try to
strike a realistic balance. This involves encouragement of a cir-
cumscribed dependence of the patient in the area of feeding and
weight, while in wider matters the therapist's role will be more that
of an uncontrolling counsellor. At times such a combination of
roles may be difficult to sustain. However, relatively simple non-
directive psychotherapy should not be thought of as a passive
technique or underestimated in its power to help people change.
Once a relationship of trust is established, the anorexic may be

able to use her sessions of psychotherapy to talk about, explore and discover thoughts and feelings which have previously been unspoken, ill defined or denied. It may be quite a new experience for her to talk with someone whom she trusts but who is not emotionally entangled with her and who, furthermore, does not overload her with advice and direction. She may come to be able to use the reflections from her therapist as a means of seeing herself and her situation in a new and more hopeful way. Psychotherapy research has defined three therapist characteristics which, in general, tend to promote a satisfactory outcome. These are the ability to empathize accurately, and to show non-possessive warmth and genuineness. Such basic characteristics may well be of value in the therapy of anorexia nervosa patients in particular and should not be beyond those practitioners who would not in general describe themselves as specialist psychotherapists.

Family psychotherapy is a logical extension of attempts to help the individual find a new adjustment. It is, of course, mainly suitable for younger patients who are living with their family of origin and for those few anorexics who are established in a family by marriage. Involvement of the family may provide the chance for everyone to examine difficulties in the past and present, but more importantly to modify the environment into which the anorexic will go in the future in such a way as to maximize her chances of full recovery. Sometimes, when the anorexic has come to occupy a place in the family which presupposes her continuing illness and dependence, the family as a whole may need help if it is to accommodate a radical change. Therapy may take the form of family meetings or sometimes of the individual support of members of the anorexic's family. For instance, a mother who has come to rely inappropriately on her sick daughter as a confidante and source of comfort in her own troubles may benefit from supportive interviews which, in turn, allow her daughter more room for manoeuvre.

Opinions vary as to when psychotherapeutic help should be given. Some authors suggest that it should be delayed until after weight is restored. While little is to be gained by such intervention if weight remains stuck at a low level, it would seem logical to begin any therapeutic relationship that is planned early in the process of weight restoration so that it is established by the time the individual is passing through the crucial stage when she is nearing a normal weight and then trying to maintain it. Likewise, there is much to be said for continuity of counselling after discharge from in-patient treatment and such follow-up may appropriately extend for a year or two, even in the absence of relapse. Recovery from anorexia nervosa may involve the appearance of other kinds of emotional disorder and these can often be understood as the result of the individual's attempts to cope differently with the problems which anorexia had kept at bay. The subject may require a variety of help. For instance, the emergence of agoraphobic behaviour might warrant both continued psychotherapy and behaviour therapy for the particular difficulty. Likewise, the emergence of evidence of profound neurotic character disorder might lead the doctor to suggest a new or an increased psychotherapeutic treatment programme.

It is clear that providing the psychological help demanded by a recovering anorexic can be a substantial undertaking for the therapist since, for the patient, the emotional transition of recovery is daunting. Any doctor who sets out to treat anorexic subjects must think how he can provide the best circumstances for this transition which his facilities, his skills and his resources allow. While there may be controversy as to which treatment regime is best, or difficulty in providing time-consuming psychological treat-ment, it would seem to be most unwise to fail altogether to consider the emotional aspects of the disorder or to plan management purely for the physical needs of the patient.

Difficult cases

It would certainly be wrong to give the impression that even the best available treatment package could be expected to be suitable for all patients, although the aims of treatment outlined above apply in most cases. But, if anorexia nervosa is viewed as a coping device, even a rather desperate one, should everyone who is an-orexic be offered treatment? The answer to this question may well be yes, but treatment and, more particularly, weight gain should perhaps not be inappropriately urged upon subjects who have been ill for many years and who have perhaps reached some kind of *modus vivendi* within the condition. This is not to say that they should not receive treatment, but rather that there are real dangers when treatment is pushed upon them too hard. There have been reports of chronically ill subjects who, having been coerced into gaining weight, have thereby lost their tenuous grip on their self-control and have committed suicide. Danger is also involved with the use of psychosurgery in the condition, although a few good results seem to have followed such operations in intractable cases. Such procedures may reduce anguish, at the expense of control.

There are special difficulties in the treatment of anorexic subjects in whom overeating and vomiting or laxative abuse have become the major problem. While standard treatment regimes are often applied to such patients, their compliance is usually less than complete and their tendency to relapse is considerable. Likewise, it is in this group of patients that some of the most severe physical complications arise. Sometimes such an individual may come to have a weight which is not greatly below normal, and may behave in some ways like a drug addict. The 'drug' in this case is food, which she consumes in vast quantities only to vomit it up again. Such a person will typically lead an active but chaotic life and her behaviour and her personal relationships will be fraught with instability. Psychotherapy in such a situation can be a difficult task for the therapist, and treatment may need to be prolonged.

Combined treatment – the story of Janet

Although this chapter has reviewed treatments aimed at weight restoration and psychological help separately, it has been emphasized that a combined approach to the problem seems to be the most rational. The following is the story of one girl's treatment. It is substantially true, although details have been changed to preserve the anonymity of the subject.

Janet was the younger child of a prosperous business man and his wife. She was aged seventeen when she fell ill with anorexia nervosa. Her background was notable in three ways. Firstly, her father worked in the food industry; secondly, her mother had had an illness in her late teens which was probably anorexia nervosa; and thirdly, mother and father lived in a state of 'cold war', both making little attempt to hide their mutual antagonism from their son and daughter. Indeed, from the age of eight, Janet had been aware of their intention to part as soon as their children had 'grown up'. As the younger child, it would be Janet's growing up that would in particular signal their ability to do so.

Janet was a tall, plumpish girl who was somewhat physically awkward and inclined to hide her marked social anxiety beneath a façade of gallumphing *bonhomie*. At the time of the onset of her disorder, she was a student at the local college of further education and was making her first tentative relationships with boys. Her activities in this sphere, as in others, tended to be characterized by an initial show of confidence followed quickly by panic and flight. After having been let down by a young man, she responded to a turmoil of self-examination and criticism by deciding she was too fat and needed to lose perhaps a stone in weight. This she did through rigid dieting, but failed to stop after losing 1 stone (6 kg) and was soon recognizably showing the features of primary anorexia nervosa. Because of her mother's history her condition was correctly identified by her parents at an early stage and the family sought the help of their general practitioner. After unsuccessful attempts to cajole her out of the condition, he referred her to a physician at the local hospital. Subsequently, when her weight had fallen to 6 stones (38 kg), Janet was admitted to a general medical ward. She remained in hospital for five weeks and was treated with chlorpromazine, some restriction of activity and encouragement to eat. During her stay she ate a little at first, but finally consumed very considerable amounts of food, and was discharged when she had put on about 20 lb (9 kg). At this time, she was determined to recover, but within days of her discharge she was again losing weight, and after a couple of months she had lost all the ground she had gained. She was now staying at home all day every day and the supervision of her eating, such as it was, had become a full time preoccupation for her mother. Indeed, faced with their daughter's illness, both parents were active and united in their common concern to help her. They discussed Janet's relapse with their family doctor and, in view of the failure of the physical approach, decided that they would seek help privately from a psychiatrist. Following assessment by the psychiatrist, Janet entered into twice-weekly psychoanalytically orientated psychotherapy which continued for the next six months. Janet disliked the therapy sessions and would sometimes refuse to go; finally she rebelled consistently and the treatment was terminated. She was still the same low weight and the family was even more demoralized. Eventually the family doctor sought an appointment with a psychiatrist with a special interest in anorexia nervosa at a London teaching hospital. An out-patient assessment, where Janet and her parents met with the psychiatrist and a social worker, lasted for a whole afternoon, but ended with an informal treatment contract being reached. Two or three weeks later, Janet was admitted to a psychiatric unit where three other young people with the disorder were already under treatment. The regime to which she had agreed included strictly enforced bed rest, a rigid expectation that she would eat the ward diet of 3,000 calories which was provided and the knowledge that she would remain on this regime until she had reached the weight of 8 st. 12 lb (56 kg), which was the strictly average weight for someone of her age and height. Although no drugs were prescribed at the outset, a moderate dosage of chlorpromazine was added for a few weeks when she found the restriction on her activity too irksome. At first Janet was nursed in a side ward, but later she was moved into the main ward when her room was needed for a 'new girl' who also had anorexia nervosa. Throughout her stay in hospital, Janet had two one-hour discussion sessions per week with a junior psychiatrist and was also included in the family meetings which took place with both psychiatrists and the social worker every two or three weeks. In spite of her agreement to the terms of treatment, it was several days before Janet settled fully into the regime, but when she had done so her progress in terms of weight gain was steady. As the weeks went by, she felt herself to be bloated and fat, and inwardly upset in a way she found difficult to put into words. Nevertheless, the formal discussion sessions provided a setting in which she could try to voice her thoughts and, most of all, the atmosphere created by the nurses and, not least, the other patients enabled her to stick to the task. However, on one occasion she got as far as packing her suitcase, but was persuaded to stay. After ten weeks she reached her target weight and was gradually allowed to get up until, after another two weeks, her activities were unrestricted. Meanwhile her diet was adjusted and after a further two weeks she left hospital for a weekend at home. By this time she felt somewhat more settled in general and in particular was getting used to her weight. Her abdomen, which at first had felt uncomfortably protruberant, now flattened off as her newly laid-down fat redistributed itself. After sixteen weeks in hospital, Janet was discharged but continued to have regular meetings as an out-patient with the junior psychiatrist who had been her therapist in hospital. Their meetings continued with decreasing frequency over the next eighteen months until he moved to another job. During that time two further family meetings were arranged when some special issue seemed to demand discussion, and Janet's mother remained in contact with the social worker. All in all the year following her hospital admission was a time of considerable emotional turmoil, and at times Janet experienced marked anxiety symptoms which for a few weeks she attempted to 'treat' by drinking alcohol quite heavily. After a 'false start' when she returned to college, she then settled into a job in a department store and began to rebuild a social life after over two years of illness. Her weight remained at, or indeed, slightly above her hospital target weight and apart from one brief spell of a few days when she overate, her diet was satisfactory. Her periods returned three months after her discharge from hospital. Two years after admission she was still a markedly nervous young woman, but had matured considerably, and showed no sign of relapsing into anorexia nervosa. She was discharged from out-patient attendance, but was told that she could contact the service again if she felt things were not going satisfactorily. Interestingly, her parents did not part and indeed seemed to have sustained a somewhat warmer relationship since their daughter's illness.

This is the story of the successful use of a treatment regime combining attention to both the physical and psychological aspects of the disorder. It was chosen as an illustration of what seems to be a good approach to treatment, but, of course, such an approach also has its failures.

The outcome of treatment

The proper assessment of the effect of treatment interventions in anorexia nervosa would demand base-line information which is not available, together with comparative studies of a kind which have not been carried out. Thus, as has been discussed previously, the course of untreated anorexia nervosa is by no means clear, even when problems raised by the definition of the disorder have been tackled. Different authorities use different criteria for measuring improvement or recovery, and different treatment centres may well have patients of different severity referred to them. Doctors who have a reputation as experts in this field may perhaps treat their patients better, but may have more difficult cases referred to them. Doctors who see anorexic patients only occasionally rarely report their results. Ideally, the treatment regimes of similar patients treated in the same centre perhaps at the same time should be compared. In practice, centres usually develop their own treatment programmes because they believe them to be the best and then apply them to all their patients. If regimes are changed this tends to be by slow evolution. As in most of medicine, the rigour of the comparisons used in such non-drug treatment rarely approaches that of modern drug trials.

Weight is an easily measured and reliable index, and it can be said with confidence that most in-patient treatment programmes lead to weight increase in their patients. Rates of increase of 7 to 9 lb (3 to 4 kg) per week have been reported, although a more average figure would be between 2 and 5 lb (1 and 2·5 kg) per week. Clearly the rate of weight increase will depend substantially on how much the anorexic eats, which in turn will be related to how much she is allowed or expected to eat. As discussed above, there are reasons for doubting that the most rapid weight gain and the biggest diet are the best plan in the long run. A better index might be the highest weight reached but, again, comparability is confounded by differences in the amount of weight gain which is attempted. Thus some centres concentrate on reaching a fixed target weight which is usually the average weight for the subject's age and height, while others are more flexible. One recent study comparing traditional nursing techniques with a behavioural programme used in the same hospital at a different time came out in favour of the latter as leading to a more rapid weight gain (Wulliemer, Rossel and Sinclair, 1975). However, the rate was not more than can be achieved by other means. Furthermore, a formal trial comparing weight gain achieved during five weeks of in-patient treatment with and without the use of behaviour modification failed to demonstrate a significant difference between the two treatment conditions (Eckert *et al.*, 1979). A study from New Zealand claimed that immediate outcome was improved after the introduction of a regime involving a strict target weight, a treatment contract with bed rest and psychotherapy (Fox and James, 1976). Earlier, less successful treatment at the centre had varied from the predominantly physical to the largely psycho-therapeutic, sometimes combined with behaviour therapy. Criteria for assessing results, however, were poorly defined. In general it would seem that when doctors and nurses use a regime for weight restoration in a way in which they are experienced, they will be able to help most of their patients to gain weight appropriately. Dally and Sargant suggested in 1966 that long-term outcome is little influenced by the means used to promote weight restoration.

The best criterion of the efficacy of a treatment would, of course, be the number of patients which it helped to recover fully. Here, again, problems of definition arise as the evidence mainly comes from series of patients from a number of centres which have taken a special interest in the disorder. The authors have not used a uniform selection from the possible list of criteria of recovery such as a maintained normal weight, resumption of menstruation, a settled and satisfactory diet, good interpersonal and sexual rela-tionships, and so on. There is some broad agreement between many of the series, but in the absence of much knowledge of the natural history of the untreated disorder, it is difficult to be sure whether these special centres are reporting the results of treatment regimes which are equally successful or equally ineffectual! It would be, perhaps, unduly sceptical to suppose that treatment had no effect. However, in most series the majority of patients did not recover so promptly in relation to in-patient treatment that there could be no room for doubt. Rather, perhaps, a period of intensive treatment initiates a time of change and some subjects may wobble along for some months or even years before full recovery takes place. Certainly such patients occur in every series. When, however, can one say that delayed recovery is or is not still in any sense the result of treatment? Many patients show a slow and interrupted progress toward recovery over years and this may, indeed, represent the natural history of the disorder in some cases.

Dally has reported one of the largest series of patients. He claims that 'once anorexia nervosa has developed, symptoms of one sort or another are likely to last for between three and five years. It is rare for anorexia nervosa to clear up in under three years. Patients may continually relapse and require readmission'. He also suggests that relapse in itself is of no prognostic significance and that after three to five years, 60 to 70 per cent of subjects will be maintaining a satisfactory weight (Dally, 1969; Dally and Gomez, 1979).

Two series of subjects, detailed below, have been reported recently using the same system of classifying outcome. Broadly, a 'good' outcome means a sustained normal weight and regular menstruation. An 'intermediate' outcome means a weight which is at times within normal limits with or without some continuing menstrual disturbance. Both series probably include a disproportionate number of severe or difficult cases.

In 1975 Morgan and Russell reported a series of forty-one subjects who were treated as in-patients at the Maudsley Hospital, London and followed up for at least four years. The treatment consisted of refeeding with nursing supervision and some brief supportive psychotherapy. Their patients regained on average 84 per cent of a normal body weight while in hospital. They used a complex but wide system of defining outcome, including weight, menstruation and a number of indices of personal and social functioning. Sixteen patients (39 per cent) were rated as having a good outcome, and of the rest about half had an intermediate and half a poor outcome. Two patients died, one by suicide and one from asthma.

The St George's Hospital Group (Hsu, Crisp and Harding, 1979) has written about a series of 105 female patients seen initially between May 1968 and December 1973. Between four and eight years later, three patients could not be traced and two had died, both of inanition and severe metabolic disturbance due to vomiting. Of the forty-nine subjects who had been offered and who had accepted in-patient treatment, including restoration of weight and psychotherapy, twenty-two patients (45 per cent) had a good outcome and eighteen (37 per cent) had an intermediate outcome. A further thirty-one subjects received out-patient supervision and psychotherapy at St George's Hospital and were probably less severely ill from the outset. Of these, twenty-two (71 per cent) were rated as having a good outcome. The remaining patients were only assessed at St George's and either received no treatment or were treated elsewhere.

All in all the message these reports give is neither bright nor hopeless. A majority of patients will recover, although some will not. Of those who do recover, many will do so only after a prolonged period of instability. There would seem to be some indication that the addition of a substantial psychotherapeutic input combined with a strict restoration of weight to a normal level carries the best promise of a sustained and relatively speedy recovery. It is clear, however, that no treatment regime is satisfactory and there is room for both attempts at innovation and careful comparisons of existing treatments. The particular difficulties of the treatment of anorexia nervosa would, perhaps, suggest that specialist centres where the doctors and also the nurses can gain special experience of the disorder may have considerable advantages. Likewise, the physical and psychological components of treatment may well be more readily combined when the anorexic is under the care of a psychiatrist rather than a general physician. Most of all, perhaps, the doctor concerned should have an interest in and enthusiasm for treating this condition which can otherwise seem so difficult and depressing.

7 • Living with anorexia nervosa

Anorexia nervosa can be a lonely and desperate state for the anorexic, a nightmare for those around her and a puzzle for those who try to help. Yet there is no quick or easy way of escaping from the condition and everyone concerned must live with and through it, while struggling to do their best to get out at the other end. There are no simple rules or principles about how to cope day to day. For the individual and her family there are no real experts. Those whose professional role has led them into frequent contact with the disorder may feel certain of how to act within that role, but have rarely struggled with a weight phobia themselves or had to face an anorexic daughter of their own. They may feel able to give advice, but much of it may be relatively untested and most of it will be a lot easier said than done. This chapter will attempt to discuss anorexia nervosa from the point of view of the anorexic and her family.

Is this anorexia nervosa?

Have I got anorexia nervosa? Has she got anorexia nervosa? This must be the first kind of query. The use of the word 'got' in these questions arises from the medical way of speaking which seems to attribute an existence of a condition to a disease entity which is almost independent of the person who 'has' it. Such a way of speaking has advantages when doctors and others are trying to define the essential common features of a number of different people who nevertheless have similar complaints. It can get in the way, however, when someone is thinking about themselves or someone near to them. It can be comforting sometimes to blame a reified and named disease for an otherwise nameless sense of distress when the disease that one then accepts as one's own is of a physical kind and readily understood. Indeed, this may sometimes be the case with a mental disorder. For instance, to construe one's emotional state as a depressive illness may sometimes allow one to behave as an ill person and to seek help. Often, however, to view oneself as sick is unwelcome and carries associations and implications that are unacceptable. This is usually the case when the question of anorexia nervosa arises in the mind of a parent or of the subject herself. Indeed, for her the fact that anorexia nervosa develops as a way of coping may cause the idea of 'having' such a named disease to be dismissed as soon as it is considered. Indeed, even the question itself may seem too direct. Perhaps a better inquiry would be in what way do I or does my daughter (or whoever) resemble people who are undoubtedly in a state of primary anorexia nervosa? This may seem an elaborate circumlocution but it does enable a situation to be dissected and examined usefully. For the following discussion it will be assumed that a parent is confronting the problem of a possibly anorexic daughter. The argument would be the same for other relationships or worry about oneself, but the use of one example case simplifies the text.

In what way does my daughter resemble a person who is in a state of anorexia nervosa? She may, of course, do so in many ways which are unimportant in this context. The crucial dimensions are those of weight, menstruation, eating and attitude. Healthy girls and young women vary considerably in their weight. Weight charts can merely give an average or sometimes a notional 'ideal' weight for the age and height of the individual. Weight alone is a rather crude index of health or illness, but it is probably true to say that if a young person's weight is within 10 per cent of the average figure then it is unlikely that a serious disorder of weight exists unless there is clear evidence otherwise. (It should be noted that an individual may be in major difficulty with a predominantly bulimic disorder and remain at or near such a normal weight. Furthermore, a young woman who was formerly obese may be truly anorexic at a weight which is average or thereabouts.) On the other hand, a weight of less than 90 per cent of average does not establish a diagnosis as some people are naturally very thin. If, however, the weight is less than 85 per cent of average there is a need to question why the individual is so different from her peers. Change in weight (weight loss) needs to be considered along with absolute weight.

The cause may often be some kind of illness, not necessarily anorexia nervosa.

Is your daughter menstruating? If she is and, furthermore, she is not on the contraceptive pill or similar medication, then she is not in a state of anorexia nervosa. Once again it may be necessary to qualify this dogmatic statement by noting that some subjects in the course of anorexia may menstruate occasionally, perhaps in relation to overeating. Furthermore, it has been known for girls to pretend to menstruate or to induce bleeding by artificial means. In general, however, menstruation is reassuring; amenorrhoea is worrying. Other causes for amenorrhoea, of course, range from emotional upset to pregnancy to serious physical disease.

Thus your daughter is significantly underweight and has not had a period for six months. What further evidence is relevant to the task of strengthening or weakening the suspicion of anorexia nervosa? The answer is her attitude to weight, and that is most often revealed by her attitude to eating. To a person in a state of primary anorexia nervosa, weight matters, it seems, more than anything else. The extent to which weight matters may be a source of anxiety or embarrassment to the individual and she may seek to conceal it. Nevertheless, the way in which she chooses what she eats and the way in which she chooses to eat it, can reveal the extent to which she is *actively* avoiding a return to a more normal weight. Furthermore, weight and eating will be sensitive but interesting topics to her. She may be very keen to be involved in preparing food for others and reading about diets for herself. There is a sense in which much mental and physical energy is being expended upon the task of avoiding eating and maintaining a low weight. By contrast, people who have lost their appetite and lost weight for other reasons will, as it were, lack energy or effort in the matter of eating. The avoidance of food and weight gain in primary anorexia nervosa is purposive; as Lasegue wrote in 1873, 'Compare this with all other forms of anorexia and observe how different they are'. In practice, of course, there may be difficulty in distinguishing the enthusiastic dieter from the anorexic and clearly a borderland exists. The distinction is one of degree and of context. The young girl who studiously counts calories and avoids carbohydrates at a fairly normal weight may be at one side of the border but she will have crossed it when she is exhibiting the same behaviour after she has lost a further 10 per cent of her former weight and stopped menstruating. The commonplace behaviour of dieting will have become abnormal as the context in which it is occurring changes. For most dieters, as they lose weight and approach their goal, their determination tends to wilt. For the anorexic, new determination is mobilized as the process of weight loss and abstinence becomes invested with new meaning and significance. As at any border, it may be the direction in which a person moves when challenged that indicates the place to which they belong. The parent of the borderline anorexic has the difficult task of issuing such a challenge without the answer being unduly confused by the process of confrontation itself. The simple matter of weighing may provide a challenging situation and a following discussion may be revealing through what is said or what is not said.

Thus, weight, menstruation, eating and attitude to weight are the criteria relevant to making a judgement about whether to worry more about the possibility of anorexia nervosa. Vomiting and purgation are relevant but they are not usually evident even when they are present; they are clearly a part of eating behaviour and attitude to weight. What are not relevant in diagnostic terms are such matters as mood, other behaviour, personality and so on. These are crucial matters in the overall consideration of a person's well-being but they should not be allowed to fog the issue. Parents and others may often make such remarks as 'It's the depression that worries me, you can't expect her to eat when she is so upset', or 'She is working hard at school at present, she is just so worried about her examinations', or 'She is not the type to get ill like that, she is such a sensible girl'. Such statements may be true and may be important, but they are not relevant to the narrow question of the diagnosis of primary anorexia nervosa.

In summary, taken together, if the young woman is not menstruating and is below 90 per cent of an average weight and, furthermore, seems to be actively maintaining that position there is real cause for concern that she may be in a state of anorexia nervosa. The lower the weight, the greater the worry. Such criteria are fairly clear, and when applied should be reassuring in some instances, raise worrying doubts in others and make a diagnosis of the disorder almost certain in some cases. The provision of such a cold list of criteria, however, may seem to suggest that resolving uncertainty is usually a simple matter for a worried parent. This is far from the case. For many reasons, the matter will be an emotional one and parents, as well as the subject herself, will rarely act in a way that is guided by reason alone. It is often remarked that those closest to the anorexic may seem to be among the slowest to see the state for what it is. As has been mentioned in previous chapters, the anorexic illness of the daughter may sometimes clearly interlock with psychological problems of the parents. However, even when this is not the case, to acknowledge that one's daughter has anorexia may carry the flavour of failure as a parent or a sense of loss of an image of her as a near-ideal daughter. It is natural to postpone the painful acknowledgement of trouble until reality forces a readjustment. Paradoxically it may seem to the parent that even to think in terms of a problem may increase the chances of it occurring and the temptation to close the eyes and hope is very real. Nevertheless, sooner or later parents will need to take the plunge and admit to themselves that there is a major problem. Only then will they be able to help their daughter.

Taking the plunge

The above discussion of lay diagnosis has been presented from the viewpoint of the parent of a possibly anorexic daughter. What has been said also applies when the situation is viewed through the eyes of the possible anorexic herself. The criteria can be used in the same way, but the task of self-scrutiny and self-diagnosis is likely to be even more fogged by self-deception and side-tracking. Having recognized and accepted that a problem exists, the subject and those close to her must decide what to do about it. Sometimes the individual may start a long, hard struggle to overcome her weight phobia without either help or disclosure of the problem to others. Sometimes such a struggle will be successful. More commonly, however, it is those near to the anorexic who first openly construe the state as a problem and raise the subject of change. As was discussed in earlier chapters, the anorexic characteristically considers her state either as advantageous or, perhaps more commonly, in a markedly ambivalent way. The prospect of change is frightening,

or at least viewed with mixed feelings. If, for instance, parents raise
the question with their daughter the initial response will be one
of denial and often hostility. As was hinted at above, such a confrontation may provoke behaviour which tends to confirm (or
deny) the suspicion of anorexia nervosa. The manner of discussion
will depend upon the people involved, the style of their usual
communication and the emotional temperature. Probably a warm
approach is best, but the topic may well prove to be a hot one!
It is in the handling of matters such as these that the so-called
expert will feel well out of his depth, although this may not
stop him feeling able to be critical after the event when things
have gone wrong! Parents in this situation cannot win, but they
can avoid losing too much. They must avoid undue procrastina-
tion.

There is a major problem and something needs to be done. But
what? Anorexia nervosa is an illness which can have very serious
implications for health or even life. Surely, if the presence of such a
disorder is suspected the answer must be to seek medical help at
the earliest possible moment. This is undoubtedly so where the
subject and her parents have reached some measure of agreement
about the problem and they have a doctor whom they know and
trust and to whom they can turn. Often, however, all parties may
feel a considerable reluctance to take this course of action. They
may feel far from certain that their diagnosis is correct and may
not wish to appear foolish or to be seen as worrying unnecessarily.
They may feel wary of putting themselves into the hands of a
doctor who might turn out to be critical and scornful of an illness
which can be so easily construed as in some way the fault of the
subject or her family. What if the doctor is sympathetic, but re-
commends methods of management which seem frightening or inappropriate? What if he starts probing and poking into the family
secrets? Surely a simple matter of not eating can be sorted out
within the family? May not creating too much fuss mean the risk of
rocking the boat and making matters worse? These are the kind of
thoughts that can lead a family to be slow to seek medical help
even after the problem of anorexia nervosa is suspected. Can such
delay be justified? The answer must arise from a balance of advantage and risk. It would be simple and safe to say that professional
help should always be sought as soon as possible, but there may be

circumstances where this may not inevitably be the only course of action. There are circumstances, however, where to wait would be clearly inappropriate or even dangerous. If vomiting or laxative abuse are evident parts of the picture medical assessment is of great importance since such complications can quickly lead to physical decompensation. Weight loss of 15 per cent or more of average weight should also indicate that help is required urgently. In general, and without other complications, real physical distress is likely when the weight falls much below this level and a weight loss in excess of 35 per cent may be life-threatening. Of course, any cause for serious concern about the physical health of the anorexic is a reason for consulting a doctor without delay. Likewise, if the personal and social adjustment of the individual has already broken down there is little to lose and much to gain from seeking help sooner rather than later. Furthermore, as time passes an anorexic tends to become more stuck within her condition and her healthy development will not be progressing smoothly. There can be little rational justification for avoiding competent help if the disorder has already been present for more than three or four months. An attempt to escape from the disorder without professional involvement would, therefore, seem to be justifiable only when the disorder is newly present in a mild, borderline or doubtful form and when there are real reasons for reluctance about seeking help. How often unaided recovery actually happens is not known, but certainly failure to recover after weeks rather than months must be added to the list of criteria for calling upon help from outside the family. Although it may be a view full of professional bias, it would seem most reprehensible to 'sit on' a severe, deteriorating or simply 'stuck' case of anorexia nervosa for long without calling upon appropriate people to join in the struggle. The dangers of complicating and exacerbating the situation through delay are very real.

In mentioning success and recovery, a word of caution is necessary. Recovery must be judged in terms of the reversal of the three criteria of illness which were discussed above. The most measurable and the most important of these is body weight. Unless weight has been restored to a normal level, recovery has not occurred. Weight restoration is a necessary although not sufficient condition of recovery. Doctors who frequently deal with anorexic patients and their families become used to such remarks as 'I'm so much better in myself and I am eating very well, although my weight is the same'. Such a statement must not be used as an index of true progress.

Eating

Whether or not there are professionals involved, most of the eating and attempts at eating of the struggling anorexic will take place at her home or at least outside of the range of professional supervision. Furthermore, although anorexia nervosa is basically a disorder of weight, the struggles and conflicts with others will usually take place around the matter of eating. Sometimes each mouthful will become the subject of discussion and negotiation, and for the individual every bite may be a battle with herself which a part of her will inevitably lose. On the one hand, the demands of her hungry body, and her former experience of appropriate eating will push her towards food. These inner feelings will be reinforced by the persuasion of others. Working in the opposite direction will be the force of her phobia of normal weight and her fear that were she to begin to eat she would be unable to stop. She fears becoming out of control. The battle is essentially with herself and within herself, but it may come to be fought largely with others. The parents of an anorexic girl may come to be seen as and feel themselves to be the only force which is promoting her feeding. Likewise, the anorexic feels that she is fighting with external forces rather than with her own feelings. Indeed, when the emotional problems of the parents contribute to their behaviour in this respect, she is partly correct. Willy-nilly, it may be easier in the short run to fight with others rather than to experience the full force of a conflict within oneself. In the longer run, however, an acceptance of the struggle as one's own and teasing it apart from external conflict is an essential condition for progress. Such an acceptance is usually partial and changeable, at least at first. The individual will shift from feeling mixed up to feeling persecuted and back, and those involved with her will at times seem to be her saviours and at others her tormentors. If such an alternation is added to the ambivalence of an adolescent/parent relationship the mixture is rich indeed.

When the anorexic subject is able to accept the problem as her own, her task will be to borrow strength and control from those around her. They should be recruited on the side of her desire to eat more normally and to gain weight. People may be effective in this role to the extent that they are seen as trustworthy and reliable, not as feeders but as controllers. The anorexic may agree to start eating if she feels others will stop her should her nightmare – being unable to stop – come true. The parents or other helpers need to keep this in mind and avoid giving the impression that the more the anorexic eats the better pleased they are. While cajoling may be necessary, it is too easy to try to tempt a starving child with all manner of sweetmeats and luxury foods in seemingly unlimited quantities. Such temptation may simply underline the subject's sense of the dangers of giving in. Somehow, in the face of the anorexic's self-starvation those around her must sympathize with her and be reassuring about her fear of eating too much. A diet composed solely of favourite and special foods can reinforce a fear of gross self-indulgence and loss of control. A run-of-the-mill diet including carbohydrates such as bread, rice and potatoes needs to be offered. Furthermore, while long-term preferences should, of course, be respected, it is best to pay little heed to new food fads which have arisen in the context of the disorder. The difficult task of the helpers is to maintain a clear and resolute expectation of 'normal' eating of 'normal' food. This may be difficult if for any reason their own eating behaviour is eccentric.

The anorexic subject needs to increase her sense of personal control over her eating. Those about her should try to bolster this sense of control even while they encourage eating. Eating has to be gradually separated from the other issues with which it has become entangled. The manner in which this goal is pursued may differ widely according to circumstances. It may often be appropriate to attempt to 'normalize' eating behaviour in a clear way, for instance, by encouraging the individual to eat at general mealtimes and to avoid nibbling at other times. Again the temptation may be to try to maximize intake by encouraging eating at any time. Such a 'little but often' style or even picking at continuously available food may be justified by such statements as, 'Her stomach has shrunk and just won't take any quantity of food at one sitting', or 'You can't expect her to eat normal meals in her condition'. In general, these tactics are inappropriate. In the short term they may increase the amount of food that is eaten somewhat, but in the longer run it may be more important to restore the style and the circumstances of eating towards a more normal pattern. To do otherwise is to risk introducing even more complication rather than simplifying and detaching eating and weight from their already overloaded emotional context.

In order to put eating in its place, it may be helpful for the anorexic and her family to be unusually deliberate and organized about eating. Within the disorder, the kind of 'automatic pilot' which usually regulates food intake has broken down and once the direction and destination have been agreed upon it will be necessary to pay a great deal of attention to the controls. Such devices as the keeping of definite mealtimes, recording and calorie counting can be useful. Anorexic subjects are often expert calorie counters and such expertise may seem to be part of the illness. However, it can be mobilized as part of the cure, if upper and lower daily limits are set realistically. Likewise, agreed rules may be useful about the discussion of food, eating and weight, so that these topics are, on the one hand, usefully aired but, on the other, are prevented from becoming the sole topic of conversation. A family with an anorexic daughter may decide to set aside half an hour each day for such discussion, perhaps after the evening meal. In this situation, argument or even conversation about these matters would be frowned upon at other times. Likewise, weighing and preparing food for others are acts which may benefit from agreed control. In a household with an anorexic member, eating and weight cannot be unimportant or neutral topics. Ignoring them or paying them little attention in the hope of lessening their importance will almost certainly fail. It is best, therefore, to try to organize the attention in such a way as to stand some chance of making matters better rather than worse.

There is no doubt that all the above suggestions are much more easily said than done, both for the anorexic and her family. The conflict within the individual can readily become a battle within the family for reasons arising both from the problems of the anorexic and those around her. It is no easy task to cope with a person who resolutely refuses to be fed, especially if the person is one's own child. It is often the case that the situation touches upon sore and vulnerable areas in the parent's own emotional make-up or aggravates interpersonal difficulties within the family. It is necessary for the parents to try constantly to separate eating and emotion and to avoid joining battle for their own personal reasons. Exasperating though the whole thing may become, such remarks as 'Your mother has spent hours preparing your favourite dish and you haven't touched it', or 'Why do you throw my food back at me?' are likely to make matters worse rather than better.

Frequently the task will prove almost impossible and the struggles of the family will simply increase the tangles. Then the anorexic will need to borrow her external control and supervision from others who are less emotionally involved. Hospital admission is often required but hospitals contain little special magic. The principles remain the same.

Seeking help

In the United Kingdom entry to all the services of the National Health Service is via the general practitioner or family doctor. This system has many advantages. The doctor is able to manage the majority of difficulties himself and the patients are able to get to know their doctor. Furthermore, the doctor is able to refer some patients for specialist opinion or management, making use of both his knowledge of the patient and of local services. It is, therefore, to her family doctor that the anorexic will usually turn for help. As was stated in the previous chapter, professions other than medicine may have much to offer in helping people with anorexia nervosa. Their role may indeed be central, although some medical involvement is desirable in a disorder with such clear physical consequences. (However, access to such skills as those of the clinical psychologist, dietician or psychiatric nurse is also by way of the general practitioners in the first instance.)

It may take a good deal of courage to go or allow oneself to be taken to the family doctor about such a matter as suspected anorexia nervosa. It involves a kind of self-exposure which is usually painful and tends to be avoided. It is not surprising that when the individual presents it may be a presentation of a part rather than the whole difficulty. Furthermore, it would be foolish to deny that some doctors are seen as more approachable than others. Sometimes it may be more difficult to approach a doctor who is something of a family friend than it would be a stranger. Sometimes a doctor who is not known may be invested with all kinds of fearful properties and opinions. Sometimes, indeed, the doctor is known to have little sympathy with disorders which are seen as of psychological origin. Nevertheless, the anorexic has little choice but to turn to her family doctor. Usually her reception will be more accepting and appropriate than her fantasies had led her to believe likely.

Having made an initial assessment, the doctor will decide upon some plan of action. He may manage matters himself or he may refer the anorexic to a local specialist. He will sometimes know of a local consultant, a psychiatrist or sometimes a physician who takes a special interest in the condition. The previous chapter was concerned with the variety of treatment approaches which may be advised in primary anorexia nervosa. The present chapter will not cover the same ground again but rather will discuss some possible reactions to treatment by the anorexic and her family.

Living with help

To become a patient is to put oneself within the influence of a doctor or a team of doctors and others about whom one has little knowledge, at least at first. It is something of a leap of faith. Ambivalence is rather characteristic of anorexic subjects; in particular, the ambivalence of attitude towards recovery from the condition. Such mixed feelings will inevitably colour the early relationship between the anorexic and those who are trying to help her. The evolution of this ambivalence is crucial. As with parents and others, the doctor will do well to avoid engaging in a battle with the patient since failure to do so may allow the anorexic to shelve her internal conflict and her own positive feelings about change and to feel wholeheartedly and determinedly at odds with an outside force. Ideally, the relationship between the anorexic and her professional helpers should be one of partnership in the task of sorting out her bodily health and internal conflict and sometimes the troubles of her family also. Both doctor and patient should consciously try to avoid an exaggeration of the 'them and us' configuration. Inasmuch as military metaphors can be justified, the battle should be within the person, and the helpers should act as allies of the more positive aspects of the anorexic. Within this struggle, eating may be construed as tactics, weight change as strategy and personal readjustment and stability as the war.

Whatever treatment plan is agreed upon, things may go well. Progress will probably not be smooth, but events will have a certain momentum. There will be hope and confidence. It is probably more useful to think in terms of a struggle giving way to personal growth and development than to talk in terms of cure. The period of recovery is certainly longer than that following the cure of most acute illnesses. However, people do recover from anorexia nervosa in relation to treatment. Things are not always complicated. A family may emerge from the anorexic illness of a member to enjoy a new stability from which vantage point the disorder seems an unreal and still puzzling nightmare. At least one family has celebrated the first menstrual period of their recovering daughter with an informal champagne party! If the emphasis of this chapter seems to be upon difficulties and negative feelings arising in relation to treatment, this should not be taken to imply that even this aspect of the experience of the anorexic is always or even often bad. The relief of engaging in treatment and the rewards of progress are real and common. The emphasis arises rather from the practical argument that it is likely to be more useful to discuss difficulties of treatment. Success and plain sailing do not require much comment. Nevertheless, even success and progress may have their difficult parts. Thus, parents who have been struggling for months may view with mixed feelings the compliance of their daughter when she is admitted to hospital. They may feel themselves to be failures and may even experience anger towards their daughter for exposing their impotence. The treatment team may seem to be succeeding at the very task in which the parents have failed. However, such a view is false since the nature of the relationship with the anorexic person is so different. Nevertheless, such a rivalry between parents and staff can occur. It will be compounded if the professionals explicitly or implicitly blame the parents. They may well already feel guilty and little is to be gained if the professionals foster that guilt or push them into a position of bitterness or resentment.

Parents who are on the defensive are unlikely to be able to work at their part in helping their daughter. On their side, doctors and others can all too easily cope with the potentially rivalrous aspects of their relationship with the parents of their patient by a retreat into ostentatious expertise. But the emphasis on 'we know best' carries the implication that 'you know nothing'. Not surprisingly, faced with such a perceived attack, parents may often react with anger or may be uncooperative. Sometimes, however, a passive–aggressive stance may occur where the parents abdicate responsibility for their daughter to 'the experts' but then bombard them with questions outside the narrow range of their expertise. 'What do you think, doctor?' can be an effective weapon against a doctor who has strayed or been pushed into territory where he is not at home. When such rivalry develops and is not coped with adequately it is inevitably the anorexic who suffers.

But what if things go badly from the outset? This will usually be because of a mismatch of expectation, attitude or goal between the anorexic and her family and their doctor. The sources of disagreement and conflict within the anorexic have been discussed above. Clearly her ambivalence about change may complicate treatment plans. Furthermore, the treatment plan presented by the doctor may be at odds with the anorexic's view of herself. The same may be true of her family. For example, the doctor's view of anorexia nervosa as a psychiatric disorder may not be acceptable. The idea may conjure up images of madness and modes of management which are rejected out of hand. 'It is not really a psychiatric illness. She is quite normal, she is not mental.' Thus parents may express their fear that their daughter is about to be classified with a stigmatized and rejected group. Many towns have a psychiatric service which is based on a large mental hospital built in the last century whose very name carries associations which are upsetting. People who have never entered such a hospital will nevertheless describe it as a 'horrible place'. Its image will be set by the distant view of a few chronically mentally ill patients who may be seen wandering near it. While it must be acknowledged that not all psychiatric hospitals are of a high standard, in general such preconceptions of psychiatry are understandable but mistaken. The majority of people who are seen by psychiatrists are not 'mad'. Psychiatry is a wide-ranging speciality. As has been suggested above, anorexia nervosa is a disorder which is well within this range. Parents and others who find themselves reacting negatively to the very thought that their anorexic relative should see a psychiatrist or enter a psychiatric hospital would perhaps do well to examine their own motives. It is easy for them to enter into a collusion with the anorexic and end up supporting her in her own denial and avoidance of confrontation with real emotional problems. If they feel that they are in receipt of inappropriate medical advice, their first recourse perhaps should be to scrutinize their own feelings carefully. Discussing the matter with a detached third party might be helpful. However, it is usually possible to arrange a second medical opinion in cases where real dissatisfaction, disagreement or doubt remain.

A major problem occurs where an anorexic resolutely and persistently refuses help. This happens perhaps less often than might be expected, but nevertheless it is not an uncommon situation. There is no easy answer. It would seem best to confront the undoubtedly frightened and desperate individual repeatedly with both a realistic appraisal of her situation and genuine but uncompromising prospects of help. Again to enter battle or to use scaring tactics is usually inappropriate and ineffective. The anorexic will finally shift her position if it seems to her that the balance of advantage and disadvantage makes acceptance of treatment a 'risk' worth taking. Sometimes an entrenched individual can be enabled to make a truly positive choice when those about her 'back off' for a while and give her psychological 'space'. Nevertheless, in a few cases increasing physical risk coupled with complete intransigence may justify compulsory intervention which, in the United Kingdom, would involve use of a section of the Mental Health Act (1983). However, the circumstances in which such a course would be considered seriously are rare and almost always compulsion can be avoided.

It may sometimes seem to an anorexic and her family that the disorder has taken over their lives. Furthermore, it may seem that its treatment and those responsible for it have also taken over their lives. They may yearn for the good old days when eating and weight were simple issues and psychiatrists and social workers were professionals who saw other people. The road to recovery can be long and tedious. It may be easy for those travelling along it to blame those who have joined them on the way. The treatment of anorexia nervosa cannot follow a single route which leads predictably to success. There will be disappointments. It is best to travel in hope, but to expect a long journey.

In many difficult states of disease or disability people may find comfort in the reassurance of the company of fellow sufferers. Anorexic Aid, a self-help organization, has a number of branches around the country. Its activities would seem to vary from branch to branch. They may include both social and supportive group meetings as well as contact over the telephone. It is difficult to be sure how effective or useful it is in practice although the idea would seem sound. Another organization, Anorexic Family Aid, is based in Norwich, England, and aims to provide support for both sufferers and their families. It also runs a national information service. (See *Further information* on p. 126 for the addresses and telephone numbers of these organizations.)

Getting better

In getting better, an anorexic must put on weight and undergo a change in behaviour and attitude. If female she must resume menstruation. Furthermore, she must find new ways of coping with herself and her life. Weight is easy to measure. Attitude and eating behaviour are less easily defined. Spontaneous and regular menstruation provides a good index of recovery when it occurs. Sometimes menstruation may take many months to return, even when the subject's weight and diet are satisfactory. However, given time the periods will almost always start again. There is little need for investigation or intervention for at least a year. Many young women greet the return of their monthly cycle as a signal of recovery and resist any idea that it should be artificially hastened. They would rather 'do it themselves'. Cyclical abdominal discomfort and other 'menstrual' symptoms may precede the return of actual bleeding by several months. Sometimes the periods fail to return or return in an irregular way. The explanation of this probably lies in dietary disturbance which continues in spite of a reasonable weight. The diet may be either patchy and deficient in carbohydrates, or erratic and swinging between times of stuffing and times of starving.

Where overeating is a problem, obesity may follow. Then a normal weight is just a station on the way up. However, some anorexics put on substantial amounts of weight but are not fully restored to their normal range. They, too, may not restart menstruating. While precise prediction is difficult, a normal weight and a normal diet including carbohydrates can be confidently expected to lead to the return of the menses in most cases.

But what of attitude change and new ways of coping? These are difficult matters to define. Sometimes an individual may be menstruating and eating well at a normal weight and yet still seem to be preoccupied with worries about weight. Such a state will not usually last for more than a few months. It will end either with relapse or with a gradual dilution of concern about weight as other matters become more pressing. Attitude will tend to follow an individual's actual behaviour even if it does so rather slowly. Likewise, if a position of physical and behavioural recovery is maintained, albeit with effort, new ways of coping may be forced upon the individual by the very experience of the changed psychobiological position in which she finds herself. Usually the new ways of coping will be much more stable and satisfactory than the anorexia nervosa that has been left behind. Occasionally, however, the individual may resort to behaviour which is equally fraught with hazard, such as excessive drinking or drug-taking. Commonly, and understandably, recovery from anorexia nervosa heralds a time of readjustment and such change may not be easy or comfortable.

Perhaps the best test of recovery is when the individual can honestly say that, even if she wanted to do so, she feels she has lost the capacity to behave as she did during the illness. When the whole range of anorexic behaviour seems not only undesirable but alien to her present self, then she can feel that the disorder is truly behind her. For most sufferers that time will come eventually.

Average weight of adults [1]

Please note that these are tables of *average* weights and that many healthy people may be somewhat lighter or heavier. A better indication of a healthy weight may be the weight at which that individual has remained stable without eating restraint.

Height (in shoes)			Average weights in pounds and *kilograms* (in indoor clothing)							
			15–16 years		17–19 years		20–24 years		25 years +	
ft	in	*cm*	lb	*kg*	lb	*kg*	lb	*kg*	lb	*kg*
					Men					
5	0	152·4	98	44·5	113	51·3	122	55·3	128	58·1
5	1	154·9	102	46·3	116	52·6	125	56·7	131	59·4
5	2	157·5	107	48·5	119	54	128	58·1	134	60·8
5	3	160	112	50·8	123	55·8	132	59·9	138	62·6
5	4	162·6	117	53·1	127	57·6	136	61·7	141	64
5	5	165·1	122	55·3	131	59·4	139	63	144	65·3
5	6	167·6	127	57·6	135	61·2	142	64·4	148	67·1
5	7	170·2	132	59·9	139	63	145	65·8	151	68·5
5	8	172·7	137	62·1	143	64·9	149	67·6	155	70·3
5	9	175·3	142	64·4	147	66·7	153	69·4	159	72·1
5	10	177·8	146	66·2	151	68·5	157	71·2	163	73·9
5	11	180·3	150	68	155	70·3	161	73	167	75·8
6	0	182·9	154	69·9	160	72·6	166	75·3	172	78
6	1	185·4	159	72·1	164	74·4	170	77·1	177	80·3
6	2	188	164	74·4	168	76·2	174	78·9	182	82·6
6	3	190·5	169	76·7	172	78	178	80·8	186	84·4
6	4	193	—	—	176	79·8	181	82·1	190	86·2
					Women					
4	10	147·3	97	44	99	44·9	102	46·3	107	48·5
4	11	149·9	100	45·4	102	46·3	105	47·6	110	49·9
5	0	152·4	103	46·7	105	47·6	108	49	113	51·3
5	1	154·9	107	48·5	109	49·4	112	50·8	116	52·6
5	2	157·5	111	50·3	113	51·3	115	52·2	119	54
5	3	160	114	51·7	116	52·6	118	53·5	122	55·3
5	4	162·6	117	53·1	120	54·4	121	54·9	125	56·7
5	5	165·1	121	54·9	124	56·2	125	56·7	129	58·5
5	6	167·6	125	56·7	127	57·6	129	58·5	133	60·3
5	7	170·2	128	58·1	130	59	132	59·9	136	61·7
5	8	172·7	132	59·9	134	60·8	136	61·7	140	63·5
5	9	175·3	136	61·7	138	62·6	140	63·5	144	65·3
5	10	177·8	—	—	142	64·4	144	65·3	148	67·1
5	11	180·3	—	—	147	66·7	149	67·6	153	69·4
6	0	182·9	—	—	152	68·9	154	69·9	158	71·7

[1] From *Scientific Tables*, published by J. R. Geigy S.A., Basle, Switzerland.

Suggested further reading

This book was written in part because of an apparent lack of material on anorexia nervosa which was suitable for non-specialist readership, especially sufferers and their families. However, other books which are now available include:

BRUCH, H. 1974. *Eating Disorders: Obesity, Anorexia Nervosa and the Person Within.* London, Routledge & Kegan Paul

BRUCH, H. 1978. *The Golden Cage: The Enigma of Anorexia Nervosa.* London, Open Books

CRISP, A. H. 1980. *Anorexia Nervosa: Let Me Be.* London, Academic Press

DALLY, P. and GOMEZ, J. 1979. *Anorexia Nervosa.* London, William Heinemann

Further information

Anorexic Family Aid National Information Centre

Sackville Place, 44 Magdalen Street, Norwich, Norfolk, United Kingdom (tel. Norwich 62 1414)

Anorexic Aid

National headquarters, The Priory Centre, 11 Priory Road, High Wycombe, Buckinghamshire, United Kingdom (tel. High Wycombe 21 431)

References

Chapter 1

CASPER, R. C., ECKERT, E. D., HALMI, K. A., GOLDBERG, S. C. and DAVIS, J. M. 1980. Clinical importance in patients with anorexia nervosa. *Archives of General Psychiatry*, 37, 1030–5

CRISP, A. H., PALMER, R. L. and KALUCY, R. S. 1976. How common is anorexia nervosa? A prevalence study. *British Journal of Psychiatry*, 128, 549–54

DALLY, P. 1969. *Anorexia Nervosa*. London, William Heinemann

DUDDLE, M. 1973. An increase of anorexia nervosa in a university population. *British Journal of Psychiatry*, 123, 711–12

FAIRBURN, C. G. 1981. A cognitive-behavioural approach to the management of bulimia. *Psychological Medicine*, 41, 631–6

GARFINKEL, P. E., MOLDOFSKY, H. and GARNER, D. M. 1980. The heterogencity of anorexia nervosa: bulimia as a distinct subgroup. *Archives of General Psychiatry*, 37, 1036–40

GULL, W. W. 1874. Anorexia nervosa (apepsia hysterica, anorexia hysterica). *Transactions of the Clinical Society, London*, 7:22. Report of a paper read in October 1873

KENDELL, R. E., HALL, D. J., HAILEY, A. and BABIGIAN, H. M. 1973. The epidemiology of anorexia nervosa. *Psychological Medicine*, 3, 200–3

KNIGHT, S. 1976. *Jack the Ripper: The Final Solution*. London, Harrap

LACEY, J. H. 1983. Bulimia nervosa, binge eating and psychogenic vomiting: a controlled treatment study and long-term outcome. *British Medical Journal*, 286, 1609–13

LASEGUE, E. C. 1873. De l'anorexie hystérique. Translated from *Archives Générales de Médecine* in *The Evolution of Psychosomatic Concepts – Anorexia Nervosa: A Paradigm* (1965). London, Hogarth Press

MORGAN. H. G. 1977. Fasting girls and our attitudes to them. *British Medical Journal*, 2, 1652–5

PALMER, R. L. 1987. Bulimia: the nature of the syndrome, its epidemiology and its treatment. In *Eating Habits*, ed. Boakes, Burton and Popplewell. Chichester, John Wiley & Sons Ltd

RUSSELL, G. F. M. 1979. Bulimia nervosa: an ominous variant of anorexia nervosa. *Psychological Medicine*, 9, 403–8

SIMMONDS, M. 1914. Über embolische Prozess in der Hypophysis. *Archives of Pathological Anatomy*, 217, 226

Chapter 2

BEUMONT, P. J. V., GEORGE, G. C. W. and SMART, D. E. 1976. 'Dieters' and 'vomiters and purgers' in anorexia nervosa. *Psychological Medicine*, 6, 617–22

BRUCH, H. 1973. *Eating Disorders: Obesity, Anorexia Nervosa and the Person Within*. London, Routledge & Kegan Paul

BUTTON, E. J., FRANSELLA, F. and SLADE, P. D. 1977. A reappraisal of body perception disturbance in anorexia nervosa. *Psychological Medicine*, 7, 235–43

CASPER, R. C., ECKERT, E. D., HALMI, K. A., GOLDBERG, S. C. and DAVIS, J. M. 1980. Clinical importance in patients with anorexia nervosa. *Archives of General Psychiatry*, 37, 1030–5

CRISP, A. H., HALL, A. and HOLLAND, A. J. 1985. Nature and nurture in anorexia nervosa – a study of 34 pairs of twins, one pair of triplets and an adoptive family. *International Journal of Eating Disorders*, 4, 5–27

CRISP, A. H. and STONEHILL, E. 1971. Relation between aspects of nutritional disturbance and menstrual activity in primary anorexia nervosa. *British Medical Journal*, 3, 149–51

CRISP, A. H., STONEHILL, E. and FENTON, G. W. 1971. The relationship between sleep, nutrition and mood: a study of patients with anorexia nervosa. *Postgraduate Medical Journal*, 47, 207–13

DALLY, P. 1969. *Anorexia Nervosa*. London, William Heinemann

FAIRBURN, C. G. 1981. A cognitive-behavioural approach to the management of bulimia. *Psychological Medicine*, 41, 631–6

FEIGHNER, J. P., ROBINS, E. and GUZE, S. B. 1972. Diagnostic criteria for use in psychiatric research. *Archives of General Psychiatry*, 26, 57–63

GARFINKEL, P. E., MOLDOFSKY, H. and GARNER, D. M. 1980. The heterogencity of anorexia nervosa: bulimia as a distinct subgroup. *Archives of General Psychiatry*, 37, 1036–40

JANET, P. *see* WALLET

KELLETT, J., TRIMBLE, M. and THORLEY, A. 1976. Anorexia nervosa after the menopause. *British Journal of Psychiatry*, 128, 555–8

LACEY, J. H. 1983. Bulimia nervosa, binge eating and psychogenic vomiting: a controlled treatment study and long-term outcome. *British Medical Journal*, 286, 1609–13

LACEY, J. H. and GIBSON, E. 1985. Does laxative abuse control body weight? A comparative study of purging and vomiting bulimics. *Human Nutrition; Applied Nutrition*, 39(a), 36–42

LASEGUE, E. C. 1873. De l'anorexie hystérique. Translated from *Archives Générales de Médecine*, 1, 385–403 in *The Evolution of Psychosomatic Concepts – Anorexia Nervosa: A Paradigm* (1965). London, Hogarth Press

NYLANDER, I. 1971. The feeling of being fat and dieting in a school population. *Acta Sociomedica Scandinavica*, 3, 17–26

PALMER, R. L. 1979. Dietary chaos syndrome: a useful new term? *British Journal of Medical Psychology*, 52, 187–90

PALMER, R. L. 1987. Bulimia: the nature of the syndrome, its epidemiology and its treatment. In *Eating Habits*, ed. Boakes, Burton and Popplewell. Chichester, John Wiley & Sons Ltd

RUSSELL, G. F. M. 1970. Anorexia nervosa: its identity as an illness and its treatment. In *Modern Trends in Psychological Medicine*, ed. J. H. Price. London, Butterworth & Co.

RUSSELL, G. F. M. 1979. Bulimia nervosa: an ominous variant of anorexia nervosa. *Psychological Medicine*, 9, 403–8

SLADE, P. D. and RUSSELL, G. F. M. 1973. Awareness of body dimensions in anorexia nervosa: cross-sectional and longitudinal studies. *Psychological Medicine*, 3, 188–99

STONEHILL, E. and CRISP, A. H. 1977. Psychoneurotic characteristics of patients with anorexia nervosa before and after treatment and at follow-up 4–7 years later. *Journal of Psychosomatic Research*, **21**, 187–93

WALLET, M. 1892. Deux cas d'anorexie hystérique. *Nouvelle iconographie de la Salpêtrière*. Quoted by Pierre Janet in his book *The Major Symptoms of Hysteria* (1929). Extract included in *The Evolution of Psychosomatic Concepts – Anorexia Nervosa: A Paradigm* (1965), eds. Kaufman and Heiman. London, Hogarth Press

Chapter 4

BROWN, G. M., GARFINKEL, P. E., JEUNIEWIC, N., MOLDOFSKY, H. and STANCER, H. C. 1977. Endocrine profiles in anorexia nervosa. In *Anorexia Nervosa*, ed. R. A. Vigersky. New York, Raven Press

BURMAN, K. D., VIGERSKY, R. A., LORIAUX, D. L., STRUM, D., DJUH, Y., WRIGHT, F. D. and WARTOFSKY, L. 1977. Investigations concerning thyroxine deiodinative pathways in patients with anorexia nervosa. In *Anorexia Nervosa*, ed. R. A. Vigersky. New York, Raven Press

CRISP, A. H., CHEN, C., MACKINNON, P. C. B. and CORKER, C. S. 1973. Observations of gonadographic and ovarian hormone activity during recovery from anorexia nervosa. *Postgraduate Medical Journal*, **49**, 584

FRISCH, R. E. and REVELLE, R. 1970. Height and weight at menarche and a hypothesis of critical body weight and adolescent events. *Science*, **169**, 397–9

GARFINKEL, P. E., BROWN, G. M. and STANCER, H. C. 1975. Hypothalamic-pituitary function in anorexia nervosa. *Archives of General Psychiatry*, **32(b)**, 739–44

NILLIUS, S. J., FRIES, H. and WIDE, L. 1975. Successful indication of follicular maturation and ovulation by prolonged treatment with L H releasing hormone in women with anorexia nervosa. *American Journal of Obstetrics and Gynecology*, **122(8)**, 921–8

PALMER, R. L., CRISP, A. H., MACKINNON, P. C. B., FRANKLIN, M., BONNAR, J. and WHEELER, M. 1975. Pituitary sensitivity to 50 μg LH/FSH–RH in subjects with anorexia nervosa in acute and recovery stages. *British Medical Journal*, **1**, 179–82

WAKELING, A., MARSHALL, J. C., BEARDWOOD, C. J., DE SOUZA, V. F. A. and RUSSELL, G. F. M. 1976. The effects of clomiphene citrate on the hypothalamic-pituitary-gonadal axis in anorexia nervosa. *Psychological Medicine*, 6, 371–80

Chapter 5

BERGER, J. 1972. *Ways of Seeing*. BBC and Penguin Books

BRUCH, H. 1977. Psychotherapy in eating disorders. *Canadian Psychiatric Association Journal*, 22, 102–8

BRUCH, H. 1978. *The Golden Cage: The Enigma of Anorexia Nervosa*. London, Open Books

CRISP, A. H. and FRANSELLA, F. 1972. Conceptual changes during recovery from anorexia nervosa. *British Journal of Medical Psychology*, 45, 395–405

KALUCY, R. S., CRISP, A. H. and HARDING, B. 1977. A study of fifty-six families with anorexia nervosa. *British Journal of Medical Psychology*, 50, 381–95

OPPENHEIMER, R., HOWELLS, K., PALMER, R. L. and CHALONER, D. A. 1985. Adverse sexual experiences in childhood and clinical eating disorders: a preliminary description. *Journal of Psychiatric Research*, 19, 357–61

Chapter 6

BALINT, M. 1964. *The Doctor, his Patient and the Illness*. London, Pitman

BHANJI, S. and THOMPSON, J. 1974. Operant conditioning in the treatment of anorexia nervosa: a review and retrospective study of eleven cases. *British Journal of Psychiatry*, 124, 166–72

CRISP, A. H. 1967. Anorexia nervosa. *Hospital Medicine*, 5, 713–18

DALLY, P. 1969. *Anorexia Nervosa*. London, William Heinemann

DALLY, P. and GOMEZ, J. 1979. *Anorexia Nervosa*. London, William Heinemann.

DALLY, P. and SARGANT, W. 1960. A new treatment of anorexia nervosa. *British Medical Journal*, 1, 1770–3

DALLY, P. and SARGANT, W. 1966. Treatment and outcome of anorexia nervosa. *British Medical Journal*, 2, 739–93

ECKERT, E. D., GOLDBERG, S. C., HALMI, K. A., CASPER, R. C. and DAVIS, J. M. 1979. Behaviour therapy in anorexia nervosa. *British Journal of Psychiatry*, 134, 55–9

FOX, K. C. and JAMES, N. MCI. 1976. Anorexia nervosa: a study of forty-four strictly defined cases. *New Zealand Medical Journal*, 84, 309–12

GOLDBERG, S. C., HALMI, K. A., ECKERT, E. D., CASPER, R. C. and DAVIS, J. M. 1979. Cyproheptadine in anorexia nervosa. *British Journal of Psychiatry*, 134, 67–70

GROEN, J. J. and FELDMAN-TOLEDANO, Z. 1966. Educative treatment of patients and parents in anorexia nervosa. *British Journal of Psychiatry*, 122, 671–81

GULL, W. W. 1874. Anorexia nervosa (apepsia hysterica, anorexia hysterica). *Transactions of the Clinical Society, London*, 7:22. Report of a paper read in October 1873

HSU, L. K. G., CRISP, A. H. and HARDING, B. 1979. Outcome of anorexia nervosa. *Lancet*, 1, 61–5

LUCAS, A. R., DUNCAN, J. W. and PIENS, V. V. 1976. The treatment of anorexia nervosa. *American Journal of Psychiatry*, 133, 1034–8

MINUCHIN, S., ROSMAN, B. L. and BAKER, L. 1978. *Psychosomatic Families: Anorexia Nervosa in Context*. Cambridge, Mass., and London, Harvard University Press

MORGAN, H. G. and RUSSELL, G. F. M. 1975. Value of family background and clinical features as predictors of long-term outcome in anorexia nervosa: four year follow-up study of forty-one patients. *Psychological Medicine*, 5, 355–71

RUSSELL, G. F. M. 1970. Anorexia nervosa: its identity as an illness and its treatment. In *Modern Trends in Psychological Medicine*, ed. J. H. Price, pp. 131–64. London, Butterworth & Co.

WULLIEMER, F., ROSSEL, F. and SINCLAIR, K. 1975. La thérapie compartementale de l'anorexie nerveuse. *Journal of Psychosomatic Research*, 19, 267–72

Chapter 7

DALLY, P. 1969. *Anorexia Nervosa*. London, William Heinemann

DALLY, P. and GOMEZ, J. 1979. *Anorexia Nervosa*. London, William Heinemann

LASEGUE, C. 1873. De l'anorexie hystérique. Translated from *Archives Générales de Médecine*, 1, 385–403 in *The Evolution of Psychosomatic Concepts – Anorexia Nervosa: A Paradigm* (1965). London, Hogarth Press

Index

In the following index, 'anorexia nervosa' is abbreviated to 'a.n.'

FOR THE BEST IN PAPERBACKS, LOOK FOR THE

In every corner of the world, on every subject under the sun, Penguin represents quality and variety – the very best in publishing today.

For complete information about books available from Penguin – including Pelicans, Puffins, Peregrines and Penguin Classics – and how to order them, write to us at the appropriate address below. Please note that for copyright reasons the selection of books varies from country to country.

In the United Kingdom: Please write to *Dept E.P., Penguin Books Ltd, Harmondsworth, Middlesex, UB7 0DA*

If you have any difficulty in obtaining a title, please send your order with the correct money, plus ten per cent for postage and packaging, to *PO Box No 11, West Drayton, Middlesex*

In the United States: Please write to *Dept BA, Penguin, 299 Murray Hill Parkway, East Rutherford, New Jersey 07073*

In Canada: Please write to *Penguin Books Canada Ltd, 2801 John Street, Markham, Ontario L3R 1B4*

In Australia: Please write to the *Marketing Department, Penguin Books Australia Ltd, P.O. Box 257, Ringwood, Victoria 3134*

In New Zealand: Please write to the *Marketing Department, Penguin Books (NZ) Ltd, Private Bag, Takapuna, Auckland 9*

In India: Please write to *Penguin Overseas Ltd, 706 Eros Apartments, 56 Nehru Place, New Delhi, 110019*

In Holland: Please write to *Penguin Books Nederland B.V., Postbus 195, NL–1380AD Weesp, Netherlands*

In Germany: Please write to *Penguin Books Ltd, Friedrichstrasse 10–12, D–6000 Frankfurt Main 1, Federal Republic of Germany*

In Spain: Please write to *Longman Penguin España, Calle San Nicolas 15, E–28013 Madrid, Spain*

In France: Please write to *Penguin Books Ltd, 39 Rue de Montmorency, F-75003, Paris, France*

In Japan: Please write to *Longman Penguin Japan Co Ltd, Yamaguchi Building, 2–12–9 Kanda Jimbocho, Chiyoda-Ku, Tokyo 101, Japan*

A CHOICE OF PENGUINS

Metamagical Themas Douglas R. Hofstadter

A new mind-bending bestseller by the author of *Gödel, Escher, Bach*.

The Body Anthony Smith

A completely updated edition of the well-known book by the author of *The Mind*. The clear and comprehensive text deals with everything from sex to the skeleton, sleep to the senses.

How to Lie with Statistics Darrell Huff

A classic introduction to the ways statistics can be used to prove *anything*, the book is both informative and 'wildly funny' – *Evening News*

The Penguin Dictionary of Computers Anthony Chandor and others

An invaluable glossary of over 300 words, from 'aberration' to 'zoom' by way of 'crippled lead-frog tests' and 'output bus drivers'.

The Cosmic Code Heinz R. Pagels

Tracing the historical development of quantum physics, the author describes the baffling and seemingly lawless world of leptons, hadrons, gluons and quarks and provides a lucid and exciting guide for the layman to the world of infinitesimal particles.

The Blind Watchmaker Richard Dawkins

'Richard Dawkins has updated evolution' – *The Times* 'An enchantingly witty and persuasive neo-Darwinist attack on the anti-evolutionists, pleasurably intelligible to the scientifically illiterate' – Hermione Lee in Books of the Year, *Observer*

Asimov's New Guide to Science   Isaac Asimov

A fully updated edition of a classic work – far and away the best one-volume survey of all the physical and biological sciences.

Relativity for the Layman   James A. Coleman

Of this book Albert Einstein said: 'Gives a really clear idea of the problem, especially the development of our knowledge concerning the propagation of light and the difficulties which arose from the apparently inevitable introduction of the ether.

The Double Helix   James D. Watson

Watson's vivid and outspoken account of how he and Crick discovered the structure of DNA (and won themselves a Nobel Prize) – one of the greatest scientific achievements of the century.

Ever Since Darwin   Stephen Jay Gould

'Stephen Gould's writing is elegant, erudite, witty, coherent and forceful' – Richard Dawkins, *Nature*

Mathematical Magic Show   Martin Gardner

A further mind-bending collection of puzzles, games and diversions by the undisputed master of recreational mathematics.

Silent Spring   Rachel Carson

The brilliant book which provided the impetus for the ecological movement – and has retained its supreme power to this day.

FOR THE BEST IN PAPERBACKS, LOOK FOR THE

A CHOICE OF PENGUINS

Genetic Engineering for Almost Everybody   William Bains

Now that the 'genetic engineering revolution' has most certainly arrived, we all need to understand the ethical and practical implications of genetic engineering. Written in accessible language, they are set out in this major new book.

Brighter than a Thousand Suns   Robert Jungk

'By far the most interesting historical work on the atomic bomb I know of' – C. P. Snow

Turing's Man   J. David Bolter

We live today in a computer age, which has meant some startling changes in the ways we understand freedom, creativity and language. This major book looks at the implications.

Einstein's Universe   Nigel Calder

'A valuable contribution to the de-mystification of relativity' – *Nature*

The Creative Computer   Donald R. Michie and Rory Johnston

Computers *can* create the new knowledge we need to solve some of our most pressing human problems; this path-breaking book shows how.

Only One Earth   Barbara Ward and Rene Dubos

An extraordinary document which explains with eloquence and passion how we should go about 'the care and maintenance of a small planet'.

FOR THE BEST IN PAPERBACKS, LOOK FOR THE

A CHOICE OF PENGUINS AND PELICANS

The French Revolution   Christopher Hibbert

One of the best accounts of the Revolution that I know . . . Mr Hibbert is outstanding' – J. H. Plumb in the *Sunday Telegraph*

The Germans   Gordon A. Craig

An intimate study of a complex and fascinating nation by 'one of the ablest and most distinguished American historians of modern Germany' – Hugh Trevor-Roper

Ireland: A Positive Proposal   Kevin Boyle and Tom Hadden

A timely and realistic book on Northern Ireland which explains the historical context – and offers a practical and coherent set of proposals which could actually work.

A History of Venice   John Julius Norwich

'Lord Norwich has loved and understood Venice as well as any other Englishman has ever done' – Peter Levi in the *Sunday Times*

Montaillou: Cathars and Catholics in a French Village 1294–1324
Emmanuel Le Roy Ladurie

'A classic adventure in eavesdropping across time' – Michael Ratcliffe in *The Times*

Star Wars   E. P. Thompson and others

Is Star Wars a serious defence strategy or just a science fiction fantasy? This major book sets out all the arguments and makes an unanswerable case *against* Star Wars.

FOR THE BEST IN PAPERBACKS, LOOK FOR THE

A CHOICE OF PENGUINS AND PELICANS

The Apartheid Handbook   Roger Omond

This book provides the essential hard information about how apartheid actually works from day to day and fills in the details behind the headlines.

The World Turned Upside Down   Christopher Hill

This classic study of radical ideas during the English Revolution 'will stand as a notable monument to . . . one of the finest historians of the present age' – *The Times Literary Supplement*

Islam in the World   Malise Ruthven

'His exposition of "the Qurenic world view" is the most convincing, and the most appealing, that I have read' – Edward Mortimer in *The Times*

The Knight, the Lady and the Priest   Georges Duby

'A very fine book' (Philippe Aries) that traces back to its medieval origin one of our most important institutions, marriage.

A Social History of England   New Edition   Asa Briggs

'A treasure house of scholarly knowledge . . . beautifully written and full of the author's love of his country, its people and its landscape' – John Keegan in the *Sunday Times*, Books of the Year

The Second World War   A J P Tavlor

A brilliant and detailed illustrated history, enlivened by all Professor Taylor's customary iconoclasm and wit.

A CHOICE OF PENGUINS AND PELICANS

The Informed Heart   Bruno Bettelheim

Bettelheim draws on his experience in concentration camps to illuminate the dangers inherent in all mass societies in this profound and moving masterpiece.

God and the New Physics   Paul Davies

Can science, now come of age, offer a surer path to God than religion? This 'very interesting' (*New Scientist*) book suggests it can.

Modernism   Malcolm Bradbury and James McFarlane (eds.)

A brilliant collection of essays dealing with all aspects of literature and culture for the period 1890–1930 – from Apollinaire and Brecht to Yeats and Zola.

Rise to Globalism   Stephen E. Ambrose

A clear, up-to-date and well-researched history of American foreign policy since 1938, Volume 8 of the Pelican History of the United States.

The Waning of the Middle Ages   Johan Huizinga

A magnificent study of life, thought and art in 14th and 15th century France and the Netherlands, long established as a classic.

The Penguin Dictionary of Psychology   Arthur S. Reber

Over 17,000 terms from psychology, psychiatry and related fields are given clear, concise and modern definitions.

FOR THE BEST IN PAPERBACKS, LOOK FOR THE

PENGUIN REFERENCE BOOKS

The Penguin Guide to the Law

This acclaimed reference book is designed for everyday use and forms the most comprehensive handbook ever published on the law as it affects the individual.

The Penguin Medical Encyclopedia

Covers the body and mind in sickness and in health, including drugs, surgery, history, institutions, medical vocabulary and many other aspects. 'Highly commendable' – *Journal of the Institute of Health Education*

The Penguin French Dictionary

This invaluable French–English, English–French dictionary includes both the literary and dated vocabulary needed by students, and the up-to-date slang and specialized vocabulary (scientific, legal, sporting, etc) needed in everyday life. As a passport to the French language it is second to none.

A Dictionary of Literary Terms

Defines over 2,000 literary terms (including lesser known, foreign language and technical terms) explained with illustrations from literature past and present.

The Penguin Dictionary of Troublesome Words

A witty, straightforward guide to the pitfalls and hotly disputed issues in standard written English, illustrated with examples and including a glossary of grammatical terms and an appendix on punctuation.

The Concise Cambridge Italian Dictionary

Compiled by Barbara Reynolds, this work is notable for the range of examples provided to illustrate the exact meaning of Italian words and phrases. It also contains a pronunciation guide and a reference grammar.

PENGUIN HEALTH

Acupuncture for Everyone   Dr Ruth Lever

An examination of one of the world's oldest known therapies used by the Chinese for over two thousand years.

Aromatherapy for Everyone   Robert Tisserand

The use of aromatic oils in massage can relieve many ailments and alleviate stress and related symptoms.

Chiropractic for Everyone   Anthea Courtenay

Back pain is both extremely common and notoriously difficult to treat. Chiropractic offers a holistic solution to many of the causes through manipulation of the spine.

Herbal Medicine for Everyone   Michael McIntyre

An account of the way in which the modern herbalist works and a discussion of the wide-ranging uses of herbal medicine.

Homoeopathy for Everyone   Drs Sheila and Robin Gibson

The authors discuss the ways in which this system of administering drugs – by exciting similar symptoms in the patient – can help a range of disorders from allergies to rheumatism.

Hypnotherapy for Everyone   Dr Ruth Lever

This book demonstrates that hypnotherapy is a real alternative to conventional healing methods in many ailments.

Osteopathy for Everyone   Paul Masters

By helping to restore structural integrity and function, the osteopath gives the whole body an opportunity to achieve health and harmony and eliminate ailments from migraines to stomach troubles.

Spiritual and Lay Healing   Philippa Pullar

An invaluable new survey of the history of healing that sets out to separate the myths from the realities.

FOR THE BEST IN PAPERBACKS, LOOK FOR THE

PENGUIN HEALTH

The Prime of Your Life   Dr Miriam Stoppard

The first comprehensive, fully illustrated guide to healthy living for people aged fifty and beyond, by top medical writer and media personality, Dr Miriam Stoppard.

A Good Start   Louise Graham

Factual and practical, full of tips on providing a healthy and balanced diet for young children, *A Good Start* is essential reading for all parents.

How to Get Off Drugs   Ira Mothner and Alan Weitz

This book is a vital contribution towards combating drug addiction in Britain in the eighties. For drug abusers, their families and their friends.

Naturebirth   Danaë Brook

A pioneering work which includes suggestions on diet and health, exercises and many tips on the 'natural' way to prepare for giving birth in a joyful relaxed way.

Pregnancy   Dr Jonathan Scher and Carol Dix

Containing the most up-to-date information on pregnancy – the effects of stress, sexual intercourse, drugs, diet, late maternity and genetic disorders – this book is an invaluable and reassuring guide for prospective parents.

Care of the Dying   Richard Lamerton

It is never true that 'nothing more can be done' for the dying. This book shows us how to face death without pain, with humanity, with dignity and in peace.